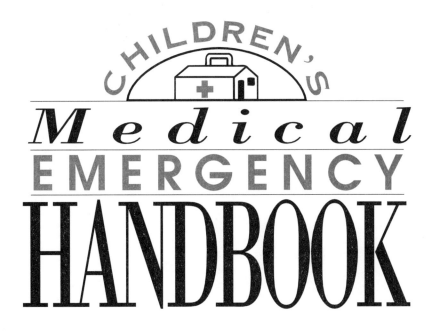

CHILDREN'S
Medical
EMERGENCY
HANDBOOK

PLUS
Over 150 Prevention Tips
And
A Special 22-Page Wellness Section

Illustrated Step-By-Step Procedures In Everyday Language
Designed By Medical Professionals
For Parents, Grandparents And Caregivers

Children's Medical Emergency Handbook
by
The Hospitals of Regina Foundation

First Printing – January 1997

Copyright© 1997 by
The Leader-Post Carrier Foundation Inc.
c/o The Leader-Post Ltd.
1964 Park Street
P.O. Box 2020
Regina, Saskatchewan
Canada S4P 3G4

Canadian Cataloguing in Publication Data

Main entry under title:

Children's medical emergency handbook

      Includes index.
      ISBN 1-895292-84-4

1. Pediatric emergencies – Handbooks, manuals, etc.
2. First aid in illness and injury – Handbooks, manuals,
etc. 3. Accidents – Prevention – Handbooks, manuals,
etc. I. Hospitals of Regina Foundation.
II. Leader-Post Carrier Foundation, Inc.

RJ370.C45 1997   618.92'00252   C97-920102-8

Cover and page design by
Yves Noblet

Illustrations by
Gail Duesterbeck

Printed and Produced in Canada by
Centax Books, A Division of PrintWest Communications
Publishing Director – Margo Embury
1150 Eighth Avenue, Regina, Saskatchewan
Canada S4R 1C9
(306) 525-2304 Fax (306) 757-2439

Introduction

In 1992, the idea of an emergency hints book was created. Although it was one of the first ideas in the very successful "Hints" book series by The Leader-Post Carrier Foundation, the book did not become a project until 1994. Under the working title of "Children's Emergency Hints", a project team was assembled. The book became *"Children's Medical Emergency Handbook"*.

The concept was simple – to provide helpful information for individuals when they needed it. Designed with the user-in-mind, the book features large print, commonly-used names, a lay-flat coil binding, simple drawings, and easy-to-understand vocabulary. The selected emergencies are those most commonly seen by emergency departments and ambulance services.

Early on, the health professionals said prevention and wellness were critical components to the book. We encourage all book purchasers to read the book and incorporate the over one hundred prevention tips into their homes. New parents and caregivers can benefit from the wellness section at the back of the book, dealing with safety and parenting issues. The "meat and potatoes" are the emergency tips that were written by health professionals and reviewed by physicians and other health professionals.

It has taken hundreds of hours from many people to bring this information together. It took longer than we thought to get the book right. When it was finished, our guiding principles – easy-to-read, easy-to-use and expert information – were honoured.

Children's Medical Emergency Handbook is a tool to help during emergencies while emergency care is being sought. No book can replace good emergency training – first aid, cardiopulmonary resuscitation (C.P.R.) – nor emergency care provided by well-trained people in our hospitals and Emergency Medical Services (EMS).

Our hope is that you will never have to use this book for an emergency. However, despite our best intentions, our children will have accidents and illness. This book is for those times.

Hospitals of Regina Foundation

The Leader-Post Carrier Foundation Inc.

LeaderPost
Carrier Foundation

The Leader-Post Carrier Foundation Inc. was established by Regina's daily newspaper as a tribute to its past and present carriers. Its aim is to support educational and humanitarian needs in Saskatchewan. While it is named in honour of carriers, help from the Foundation is available to the public at large.

Individual and corporate donations help fund the Foundation, but its primary income is from the proceeds of special projects organized on behalf of the Foundation by The Leader-Post.

Among the most successful projects have been previous books: *Money and Time-Saving Household Hints; Environmental and Energy Hints; Getting It Together; A Year of Crafts; Cornerstones, An Artist's History of The City of Regina; Work Tips: Organizing Strategies for a Productive Worklife* and *Home Tips: Organizing Strategies for a Streamlined Homelife.*

Children's Medical Emergency Handbook is the Foundation's eighth publication.

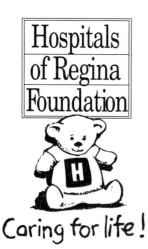

Hospitals of Regina Foundation

Caring for life!

The Hospitals of Regina Foundation was the first Foundation in Canada to raise money for all hospitals in one major centre. Initially launched with a capital campaign in 1987, the Foundation has become a permanent charitable Foundation. Its sole mandate is to raise funds to purchase equipment for Regina hospitals.

A volunteer Board of Directors, drawn from the community, sets the direction for the Foundation. Funds are raised from donations, gaming and special projects. Funds from the sale of *Children's Medical Emergency Handbook* have been designated for pediatrics and emergency equipment needs in Regina hospitals.

Regina hospitals are the base hospitals for southern Saskatchewan, providing specialized diagnostic and treatment services for a catchment area of 500,000 people. Over 200,000 patients visit the Regina hospitals annually.

Acknowledgements

Children's Medical Emergency Handbook was developed, written, and edited by many dedicated people who shared the vision of an emergency handbook written for people who care for children. While diverse specialities such as pediatrics, burns, emergency medical services, education services, family/sport medicine, community health, intensive care, emergency, adolescent, orthopedics, social work, neonatal and others were involved, the one thing every one shared was their love of children. The writers and reviewers were all volunteers, people who though so much of the idea they committed their time and energy.

Like all projects, the people involved thought it would be less work than it was. The following people, some more than others, desire our sincere gratitude;

Bruce Anderson

Bryan Barootes, M.D., C.C.F.P.

T.K. Belgaumkar, M.B.B.S.,M.D. F.R.C.P.(C.)

Barb Beaurivage, R.N.

Michelle Bilan, R.N., B.Sc.N.

Julie Briere

Glenda Coleman-Miller, R.N, B.S.N.

Peter Chang, M.D., F.R.C.S. (C.)

Sharon Chow, B.S.N.

Louise Eikerman, R.N.

Margo Embury

Tyronne Fisher, B.S.W.

Iona Glabus

Marlene Hall, R.N.

Karen Hewson, B.S.N.

Carolyn Hoffman, R.N., B.S.N., ENC (C)

Angus Juckes, M.D., F.R.C.S.(C.)

Wayne Kuss

Esther Labelle, R.N.

Joe Laxdal

Marlene Lindberg, B.H.J., M.S.A.

Jamie McMillan, R.N.

Justin Naude, M.B., Ch.B., F.C.S (S.A.), F.R.C.S. (C.)

Barbara Norum, R.N., B.S.N.

Richard Nuttall, M.B.B.S., M.D., C.C.F.P.

Jim O'Carroll, M.D.

Linda Paidel, A.P.R.

Steve Rapanos, EMT

Laura Saparlo, B.S.N.

Marcia Scott, R.N., B.S.N.

Leslie Sparling, R.N., B.S.N.

Tanya Strom, EMT-P

Joey Sweeney, R.N.

The Leader-Post – Pre Press Department

Lynn Ward, R.N.

THANK YOU!

Table of Contents

Wellness Section

Abuse: Emotional

Emotional abuse is often described as repeatedly rejecting or intimidating a child.

MAY SEE:
- sleeping problems
- fearfulness/poor self-esteem
- poor weight gain and growth
- hurting self
- behavior problems

- bed wetting
- rocking self
- eating problems
- sadness
- learning/concentration difficulties

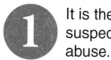 It is the law to report any suspected or known child abuse.

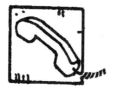 If you suspect a child is being abused, contact any of the following for guidance and more information:

- police
- crisis line
- public health nurse
- family doctor
- social services department

PREVENTION:

- Know, watch for and recognize the signs and symptoms of an abuser:
    - often were abused themselves
    - abuse alcohol and other drugs
    - feel they have no support
    - are overstressed
    - have a violent temper
    - feel out of control

- If you recognize any of these signs in yourself, call:
    - crisis line
    - social service agency
    - public health nurse
    - family doctor

- Parenting programs can often provide needed support.

- KID'S HELP PHONE: 1-800-668-6868 in Canada.

NOTES:

Abuse: Physical

Physical abuse is often described as hitting or causing harm physically.

MAY SEE:
- bruises all over or in areas not usually injured in play
- unexplained bruises or wounds
- burns/bite marks/hand marks
- behavioral changes (quiet/withdrawn)
- broken/dislocated bones
- bloodshot eyes
- weight loss
- head injuries

 It is the law to report any suspected or known child abuse.

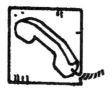

 If the abuse is currently happening, call your local police department or social services department.

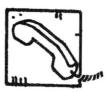 If you suspect a child is being abused, contact any of the following for guidance and more information:
- police
- crisis line
- public health nurse
- family doctor
- social services department

PREVENTION:

- Know, watch for and recognize the signs and symptoms of an abuser:
    - often were abused themselves
    - abuse alcohol and other drugs
    - feel they have no support
    - are overstressed
    - have a violent temper
    - feel out of control

- If you recognize any of these signs in yourself, call:
    - crisis line
    - social service agency
    - public health nurse
    - family doctor

- Parenting programs can often provide needed support.

- KID'S HELP PHONE: 1-800-668-6868 in Canada.

NOTES:

Abuse: Sexual

Sexual abuse may range from inappropriate touching to sexual intercourse.

MAY SEE:
- bruises/abdominal pain
- cuts in mouth, anus, private parts
- blood stain on underwear
- itching in private parts
- sudden fear of abusers or strangers
- bad smelling drainage from penis or vagina
- acting out of sexual behaviors

- bleeding
- torn underwear
- pain when urinating
- sexually transmitted disease
- venereal warts
- regressive behavior (bed wetting, thumb sucking)
- sudden change in school performance

NOTE: Believe the child and tell the child that this is not his or her fault.

 It is the law to report any known or suspected child abuse.

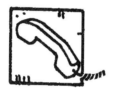

 If you suspect a child is being abused, contact any of the following for guidance and more information:
- police
- crisis line
- family doctor
- public health nurse
- social services department

 If the abuse happened recently, do not bathe the child or change the clothing so that proper evidence can be obtained.

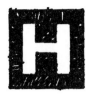 Go to your local hospital emergency department or your doctor so that proper evidence can be obtained.

5 Tell the child that this is not his or her fault and that it is safe and okay to tell the truth. Believe your child. Seek counselling for yourself and your child.

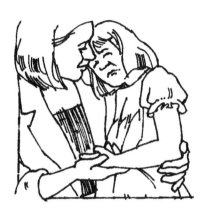

PREVENTION:
- Talk openly with your children about sexuality. Teach children at a young age what their private parts are and not to let anyone touch them.

- Know, watch for and recognize the signs and symptoms of an abuser:
  - often were abused themselves
  - abuse alcohol and other drugs
  - feel they have no support
  - are overstressed
  - have a violent temper
  - feel out of control

- If you recognize any of these signs in yourself, call:
  - crisis line
  - social service agency
  - public health nurse
  - family doctor

- Parenting programs can often provide needed support.

- KID'S HELP PHONE: 1-800-668-6868 in Canada.

Alcohol Poisoning/Intoxication

MAY SEE:
- agitation
- clumsiness
- chills
- may smell alcohol on the breath
- sleepiness
- confusion
- vomiting
- unconsciousness

 Ensure the child is breathing and has a pulse.

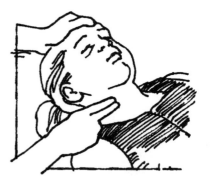

 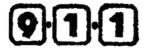 If the child is not breathing or not responsive call 9-1-1 or your local Emergency Medical Services number. Refer to:

BREATHING/C.P.R.		UNCONSCIOUS	
0 to 1 year	Page 34	0 to 1 year	Page 172
Over 1 year	Page 38	Over 1 year	Page 176

3 Keep the child on his or her side in case of vomiting.

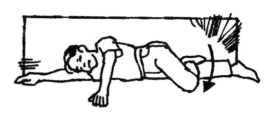

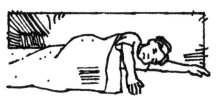 Keep the child warm and in recovery position (lying on his or her side).

5 Call your doctor or visit your local hospital emergency department. **This may be a life-threatening situation.**

PREVENTION:
- Keep alcohol, chemicals and all other dangerous substances out of the reach of children.
- Openly discuss the effects of alcohol with your children.

Allergic Reactions

MAY SEE:
- difficulty breathing, wheezing
- swelling of eyelids, lips, tongue or throat
- red skin or small, raised, red welts, hives
- sneezing or runny nose

- coughing, choking
- rapid heart rate
- itching of skin/nose
- stuffy nose

Remove the child from the suspected cause of allergic reaction.

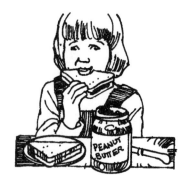

If the child has difficulty breathing or sudden and severe onset of swelling or hives, call 9-1-1 or your local Emergency Medical Services number. If the child stops breathing, refer to:

BREATHING/C.P.R.	
0 to 1 year	Page 34
Over 1 year	Page 38

Observe carefully for worsening of reaction.

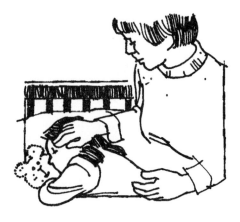

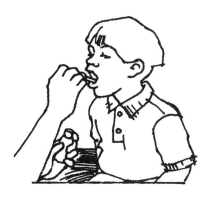

 4 If emergency care is not needed, give over-the-counter antihistamine, as directed by your doctor or pharmacist, for reducing the symptoms, and continue to watch for worsening reaction.

 5 Cold water compresses and cornstarch baths may help reduce the itching.

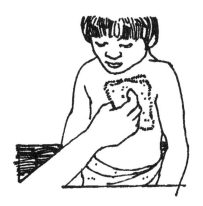

  6 Call your doctor or visit your local hospital emergency department as needed.

COMMENTS:
- If this is your child's first allergic reaction, have him or her seen by a doctor.

PREVENTION:
- Teach children to avoid things to which they are allergic.
- Children with known, severe allergic reactions should carry their prepared emergency medication (with instructions) and wear an allergy bracelet.
- Inform all teachers and care givers about allergies and appropriate emergency care.

Amputations

1 If the child is not responding or if there is serious bleeding, call 9-1-1 or your local Emergency Medical Services number. Refer to:

9·1·1

BREATHING/C.P.R.	
0 to 1 year	Page 34
Over 1 year	Page 38

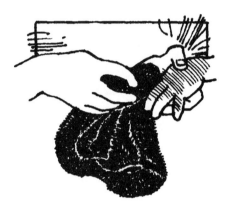

2 Apply direct pressure over the wound with your hand or a clean cloth or towel.

3 If bleeding is severe, keep the wounded area above the level of the heart.

4 If the cloth or towel on the wound becomes soaked with blood, DO NOT REMOVE IT. Place another clean cloth or towel on top and continue to apply pressure (repeat this step as necessary).

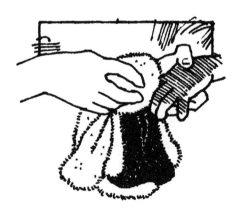

5 If the body part is still attached, stabilize it. DO NOT TEAR IT OFF.

6 If the body part is not attached, wrap the amputated part in a clean cloth and place it in a waterproof bag or container. Place the first container in a second container of ice and water.

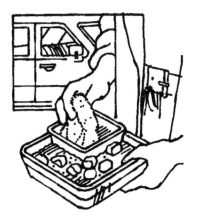

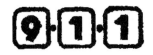

7 Call 9-1-1 or your local Emergency Medical Services number for further care or transport to the hospital immediately.

COMMENTS:
- DO NOT attempt to clean or wash the amputated part.
- DO NOT place the amputated part directly on the ice because freezing will destroy tissue.

PREVENTION:
- Keep children out of reach of mechanical and farm equipment.
- Do not leave children unsupervised.
- Teach children street, farm, tool and railway safety.

Back And Neck Injury

MAY SEE:
- pain
- tingling
- numbness
- loss of movement.

 1 DO NOT MOVE the child unless there is immediate danger or he or she is not breathing.

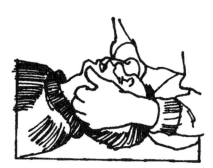

2 Check for breathing and determine if the child is awake. If the child is not breathing, refer to:

BREATHING/C.P.R.	
0 to 1 year	Page 34
Over 1 year	Page 38

If the child is not responsive:

UNCONSCIOUS	
0 to 1 year	Page 172
Over 1 year	Page 176

3 Call 9-1-1 or your local Emergency Medical Services number.

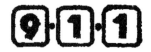

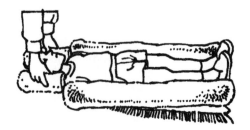

4 Keep the head and body still. Use available linen and household objects to assist you.

5 If the child or infant begins to vomit, carefully roll the child onto his or her side, keeping the head in line with the body. Clean vomit out of the mouth with fingers.

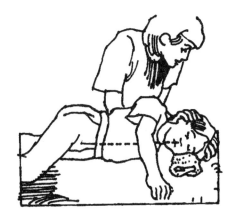

PREVENTION:

- Encourage the use of properly fitted protective sports equipment.

- Always use child safety seats or restraints correctly.

- Always supervise children at play.

- Teach children to never dive or jump into unknown waters; enter feet first.

- Teach children traffic, bicycle and playground safety.

Bites: Animal And Human

1 Apply pressure to the wound with a clean cloth.

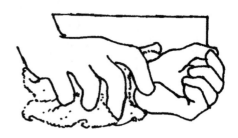

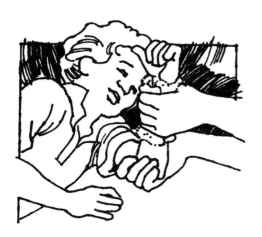

2 Keep the wounded area above the level of the heart, if bleeding is severe.

3 If bleeding is not severe, clean area with mild soap and water and cover with a clean bandage. Do not apply any creams.

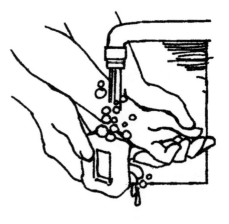

Call your doctor or visit your
local hospital emergency
department:
- immunization may be needed
- may need testing for disease
- antibiotics may be needed

COMMENTS:
- Bites can very easily become infected or spread diseases.
- Know the location of the animal or person that inflicted the bite so they can be evaluated for disease.

Bites: Poisonous Snake

1 Remove the child from danger.

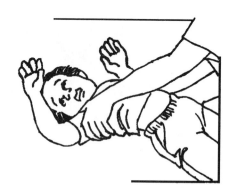

9·1·1

2 Call 9-1-1 or your local Emergency Medical Services number if the snake is or may be poisonous.

3 Watch for breathing problems. If breathing stops, go to:

BREATHING/C.P.R.	
0 to 1 year	Page 34
Over 1 year	Page 38

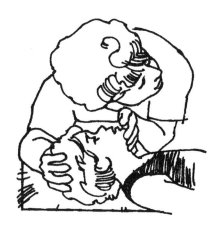

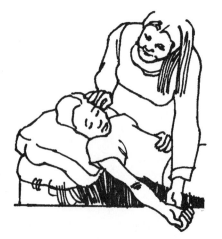

4 Keep the child warm, calm and still. Walking will spread the poison.

5 Remove any tight clothing or jewelery from the child.

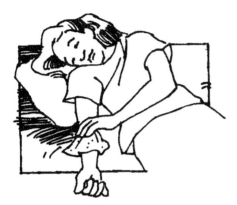

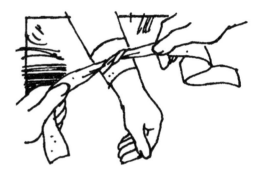 **6** Keep the area still and lower than the child's heart.

 7 If the bite is on a limb, tie a bandage or cloth above the bite. Loosen cloth if the limb becomes cold and blue.

6 Visit your local hospital emergency department.

COMMENTS:
- Remember what the snake looked like so that proper treatment may be given.
- Always seek medical attention.

Bleeding In Stools *(Bowel Movement)*

MAY SEE: • blood
• black tarry stools

1 If the child is cool, clammy, weak, pale, thirsty, vomiting blood, dizzy, faint or has a rapid heart beat, call 9-1-1 or your local Emergency Medical Services number. Refer to **Shock** on page 146.

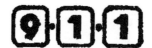

2 Do not give the child food or drink.

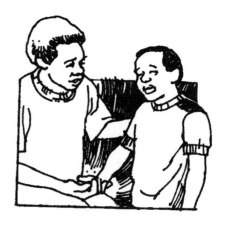

3 Comfort and reassure the child.

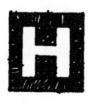

4 Call your doctor or visit your local hospital emergency

COMMENTS:

- Stools may appear black due to certain foods or medication (e.g., iron, licorice).
- Small streaks of bleeding may indicate a possible sore in the rectal area, constipation, or other bowel condition. Discuss this with your doctor or public health nurse.

NOTES:

Blisters

1 Do not break the blister. It is protecting a damaged area.

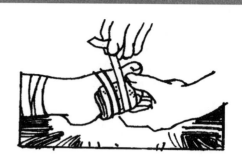

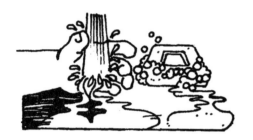

2 If the blister breaks on its own, wash the area with mild soap and water and cover it with a clean bandage.

3 If the blister is spreading or covering a large part of the body, call your doctor or visit your local hospital emergency department.

4 If the blister is red, has pus or is causing a large amount of pain, it may be infected. Visit your doctor.

PREVENTION:
• Ensure that your child's shoes fit properly and comfortably.

NOTES:

Blood Suckers And Leeches

 Put salt on the leeches if salt is available.

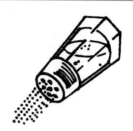

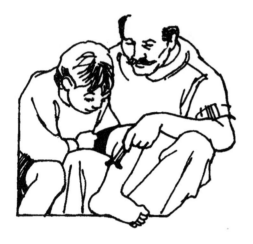

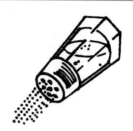 Always remove the leech and check for others.

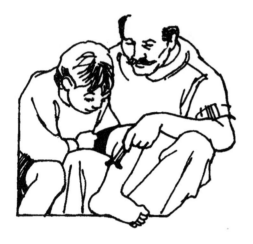 Clean the area with soap and water.

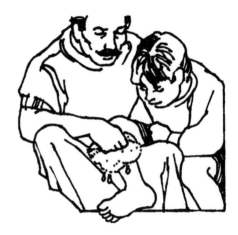

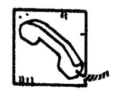

 Call your doctor if you notice a fever or rash.

COMMENT:
• Leeches usually do not cause medical complications.

NOTES:

Boils

MAY SEE: • painful red bump with a white center.

 Call your doctor if:
- the boil is on the child's face
- the child has a fever
- red streaks or more boils develop
- the boil does not break and drain on its own within a week
- the infection continues after the boil breaks.

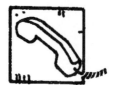

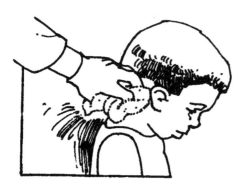

 Apply warm compresses to the boil (5 mL [1 teaspoon] of salt in 1 litre [1 quart] of warm water).

Do not force a boil open by squeezing or opening it. This action may spread the infection.

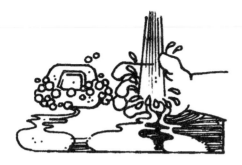

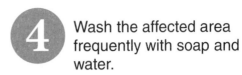

4 Wash the affected area frequently with soap and water.

5 Apply sterile bandages after the boil breaks.

COMMENTS:

- The white center of the boil will usually increase in size, break and drain in four to seven days.

- Infection is caused when bacteria enters a break in the skin. When fluid drains from a broken boil, infection may spread.

- See your doctor if skin infection reoccurs.

Breathing/C.P.R. - Infants *(Newborn To 1 Year)*

MAY SEE:
- limpness
- unresponsive (will not wake up)
- pale or bluish color
- not breathing

 Establish unresponsiveness by gently tapping the infant's feet and hands. DO NOT SHAKE.

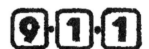 DO NOT LEAVE THE INFANT. If not responsive (not waking up) and you are not alone, have someone call 9-1-1 or your local Emergency Medical Services number.

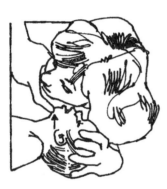

 AIRWAY
Open airway by gently tilting the head back with one hand, and lifting the chin with the other hand.

If you suspect a neck injury due to a fall or a motor vehicle accident, etc., carefully perform the chin lift to avoid twisting the neck.

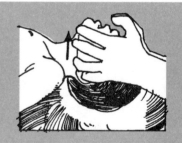

CHECK FOR BREATHING FOR THREE TO FIVE SECONDS
- **Look** to see if the chest/stomach is moving
- **Listen** for sounds of breathing
- **Feel** for air on your cheek

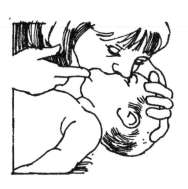

BREATHING B

5 Give two breaths of air by covering the mouth and nose with your mouth. If air does not enter with the first breath, reposition the head and try to breathe for the infant again.

DOES THE STOMACH AND CHEST RISE WITH BREATH?

NO: (If YES, turn to the next page.)

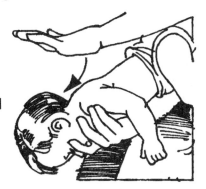

6 If the airway is blocked, give up to five back blows, using the heel of your hand, followed by up to five chest thrusts.

Chest Thrust Landmarks:
- Draw an imaginary line between the two nipples.
- Move three fingers towards the middle of the chest with your index (pointer) finger touching that line.
- Lift the index (pointer) finger and press down one-half to one inch with two fingers (you should be on the lower part of the breast bone – one finger width below the imaginary line).

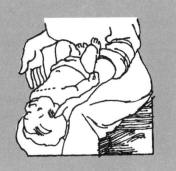

Check the airway. **Only** if you **see** the object, use your fingers to "sweep" the object. If the object is not visible, continue back blows and chest thrusts.

Continued Next Page

DOES THE STOMACH AND CHEST RISE WITH BREATHING?

YES:

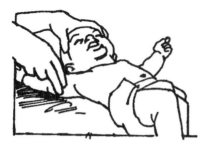

 7 **CIRCULATION** **C**
Check for pulse: (Brachial – take five to ten seconds). Place two fingers halfway between the elbow and shoulder in the middle, inside part of the arm.

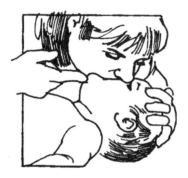

8 If the infant is not breathing but the pulse is present, start rescue breathing (one breath every three seconds or about 20 breaths per minute).

 9 **IF NO PULSE:**

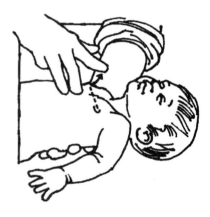

- Draw an imaginary line between the two nipples, move three fingers towards the middle of the chest. With your index (pointer) finger touching that line, lift the index (pointer) finger and press down one-half to one inch with two fingers (you should be on the lower part of the breast bone, one finger width below the imaginary nipple line).
- Press down five times (this should take about three seconds)
- After you press down five times, give one slow breath (5:1 cycle).

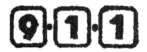 **10** If you are alone, do C.P.R. (5:1 cycle) for approximately one minute (20 cycles of 5:1). If 9-1-1 or Emergency Medical Services number has not already been called, take the infant with you and call now.

- Check pulse and breathing (three to five seconds for pulse and breathing check).
- If there is no pulse and no breathing, continue five compressions to one breath.
- Continue to check for pulse and breathing every few minutes.

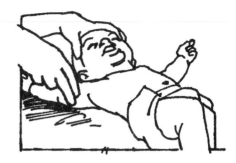

(This section was written to the 1992 CPR guidelines of the Heart and Stroke Foundation of Canada.)

COMMENTS:
- Remember your ABC's (A = Airway, B = Breathing, C = Circulation/Pulse).
- CPR is a complex skill to learn. You should enroll in a CPR class. For more information call your local community college, The Red Cross, St. John Ambulance or the Heart and Stroke Foundation.

PREVENTION:
An ounce of prevention is worth a pound of cure
- Cut food into small pieces and make sure infants or children chew food well.
- Popcorn, nuts, small candies should not be given to infants or children.
- Foods such as grapes, spaghetti, wieners, etc. should be cut into small chewable pieces.
- Infants or children should sit down to eat, never allow them to run around while eating.
- Only use pacifiers that are one piece.
- Don't hang trinkets, toys, pacifiers or necklaces around baby's neck.
- Always place infants or children in a car seat in the back seat while riding in vehicles.
- Make sure all toys have secure pieces (e.g., eyes of stuffed animals won't pull off).
- Infants or children should wear helmets while in bicycle carriers or trailers.
- Cover electrical outlets.
- Keep children away from workshop areas.
- Keep matches out of infants' or children's reach.
- Make sure all medications and/or poisons are in a safe locked place.
- Keep balloons and rubber gloves away from infants or children.
- Keep drapery strings and any cords out of infants' or children's reach.
- Do not dress infants or children in clothing with a drawstring, hood or scarf when they may be playing on play structures.
- Make sure toilet seats are down.
- Keep small, shiny objects out of infants' or children's reach (e.g., coins, earrings, marbles).

Breathing/C.P.R.: Children (Over 1 Year)

MAY SEE:
- limpness
- unresponsiveness (will not wake up)
- pale or bluish color
- not breathing

 Establish unresponsiveness: shout in both ears and pinch shoulders. DO NOT SHAKE.

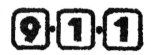 If you are not alone, have someone call 9-1-1 or your local Emergency Medical Services number.

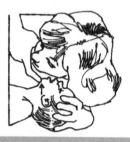

AIRWAY

Open airway by gently tilting the head back with one hand, and lifting the chin with the other hand.

If you suspect a neck injury due to a fall or a motor vehicle accident, etc., carefully perform the chin lift to avoid twisting the neck.

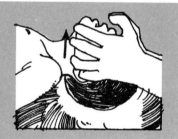

CHECK FOR BREATHING FOR THREE TO FIVE SECONDS
- **Look** to see if chest/stomach is moving
- **Listen** for sounds of breathing • **Feel** for air on your cheek.

BREATHING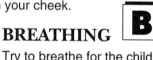

Try to breathe for the child. If the child is small, you may need to cover the mouth and nose with your mouth. Give two breaths of air:
• Keep one hand on the child's head to maintain airway. • Watch for the chest to rise and allow time for the chest to fall between breaths.

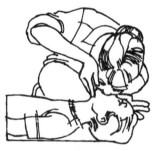

CIRCULATION

Check for carotid pulse: take five to ten seconds. Find the carotid pulse by locating the middle part of the neck and gently sliding your fingers into the groove in the neck on the side closest to you.

If the child is not breathing but the pulse is present, start rescue breathing: one breath every three seconds or about 20 breaths per minute.

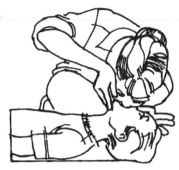

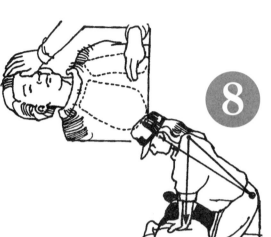

 IF NO PULSE
Run your fingers up the side of the rib cage closest to you until you reach the point where the rib cage meets. Place your middle finger there and place your index (pointer) finger next to it. Note this spot and place the heel of the bottom hand just above it. You should be on the lower part of the breast bone. Press down one to one and one-half inches.
Press down five times (this should take about three seconds).
After you press down five times, give one slow breath (5:1 cycle).

 If you are alone, do C.P.R. (Cycle 5:1) for approximately 1 minute (20 cycles of 5:1). If 9-1-1 or Emergency Medical Services number has not already been called, take the child with you and call now.

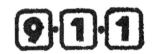

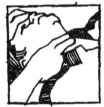 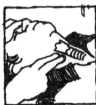 Check pulse and breathing (three to five seconds for pulse and breathing check). If there is no pulse and no breathing, continue five compressions to one breath. Continue to check for pulse and breathing every few minutes.

(This section was written to the 1992 CPR guidelines of the Heart and Stroke Foundation of Canada.)

COMMENTS:
Remember your ABC's (A = Airway, B = Breathing, C = Circulation/Pulse). CPR is a complex skill to learn. You should enroll in a CPR Class. For more information on how you can take a CPR class, contact your local community college, Red Cross, St. John Ambulance or the Heart and Stroke Foundation.

PREVENTION:
See the Prevention List on page 37.

Broken Bones

MAY SEE:
- pain
- bruising
- child will not move arm or leg
- blue color
- swelling
- bone sticking out
- tingling, numbness
- bleeding

 Keep the child safe from further injury.

 If the child is bleeding profusely, or is cool, clammy, weak, pale, thirsty, dizzy, faint, or has a fast heart beat, call 9-1-1 or your local Emergency Medical Services number. Refer to **Shock** on page 146.

3 Remove any jewellery from the limb and loosen tight clothing.

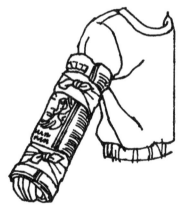

4 Try not to move the broken limb. Splint the joints above and below the injured area (e.g., use rolled towels, catalogue, cardboard, magazines, pillow).

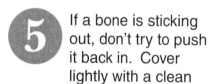

5 If a bone is sticking out, don't try to push it back in. Cover lightly with a clean cloth.

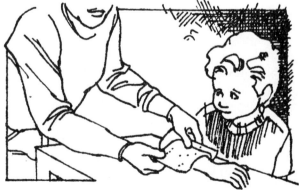

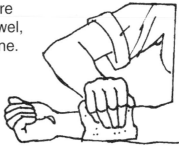

6 If bleeding, apply direct pressure to area with a clean cloth or towel, **without** moving the broken bone.

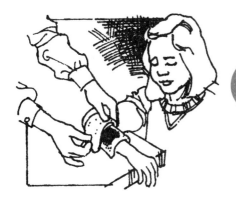

7 If the cloth or towel becomes soaked with blood, DO NOT REMOVE IT. Place another clean cloth or towel on top (repeat this step as necessary).

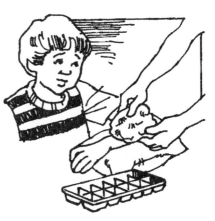

8 Apply an ice pack to the break area, except over an open wound.

9 Do not give the child food or drink.

10 Visit your local hospital emergency department.

COMMENTS:
- Accidents are the leading cause of death in children.

PREVENTION:
- Encourage the use of properly fitted protective sports equipment.
- Always use child safety seats or restraints correctly.
- Always supervise children at play.
- Teach children to never dive or jump into unknown waters; enter feet first.
- Teach children traffic, bicycle and playground safety.

Bruising

1 If your child has suddenly developed a large number of unexplained bruises, visit your doctor.

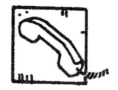

2 In most cases, bruises are caused by a bump or fall.

3 If the bruised area is also swollen, you can use an ice pack to help the swelling go down (within the first 24 to 48 hours of the injury).

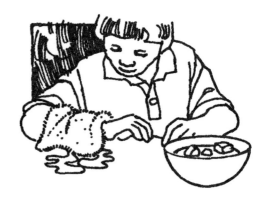

4 Bruises will fade in approximately two weeks.

5 Applying warmth to an old bruised area (after 48 hours) may help it fade faster.

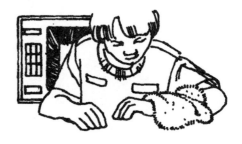

COMMENTS:

• Be aware that if the bruises are appearing for no apparent reason, it is important to see your doctor.

NOTES:

Burns: Chemicals On The Skin

ENSURE YOU ARE NOT IN CONTACT WITH CHEMICALS WHILE HELPING:
Wear gloves. Do not attemp to neutralize any chemicals.

MAY SEE:
- burning and redness of skin
- rash
- swelling
- itchiness
- blisters
- fever

 If the child is having trouble breathing or does not respond, call 9-1-1 or your local Emergency Medical Services number. Refer to:

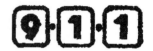

BREATHING/C.P.R.		UNCONSCIOUS	
0 to 1 year	Page 34	0 to 1 year	Page 172
Over 1 year	Page 38	Over 1 year	Page 176

 If the burns are severe, or on the child's face, call 9-1-1 or your local Emergency Medical Services number.

 If the child is unconscious, identify the chemical and call the poison control center or visit your local hospital emergency department for advice.

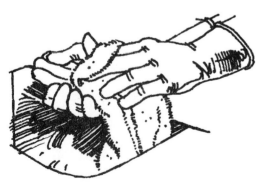

 Wearing gloves, remove any chemicals that are in contact with the skin. Use a clean, dry cloth. Throw the cloth away.

Flush the child's skin with running water for at least 15 minutes:
- Use a shower if needed
- Remove any clothing and jewelery from the child while in water
- Avoid getting the chemical in the child's eyes or mouth

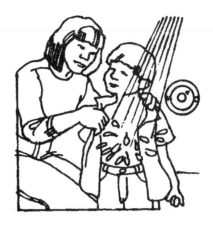

 Cover the burned area with a clean, dry cloth or bandage.

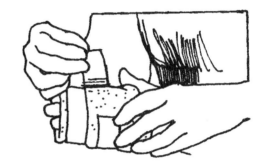

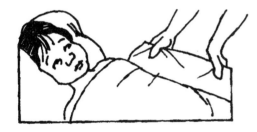

 Keep the child warm and comforted.

PREVENTION:
- Keep all chemicals in a locked cupboard, away from children's reach.
- Teach children the meaning of chemical warning symbols on containers.
- Keep the poison control number by the phone and write the number inside the front cover of this book.

Burns: Electrical

PROTECT YOURSELF. DO NOT TOUCH THE CHILD UNTIL THE POWER IS OFF.

MAY SEE: • black charring at one or two places on body or limbs

ANY OF THESE DEEP BURNS MUST BE TREATED BY A DOCTOR.

 If the child is having trouble breathing or does not respond, call 9-1-1 or your local Emergency Medical Services number. Refer to:

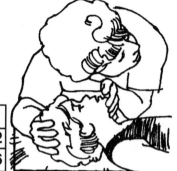

BREATHING/C.P.R.		UNCONSCIOUS	
0 to 1 year	Page 34	0 to 1 year	Page 172
Over 1 year	Page 38	Over 1 year	Page 176

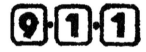 Call 9-1-1 or your local Emergency Medical Services number if:
• burns are severe or on the face
• there is a lot of smoke in the room
• the child is under two years of age
• the child is unconscious

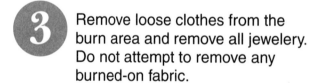 Remove loose clothes from the burn area and remove all jewelry. Do not attempt to remove any burned-on fabric.

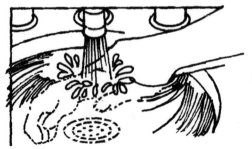 Flush burned area with room-temperature water for at least five minutes.

5 Cover the burn with a clean, dry cloth.

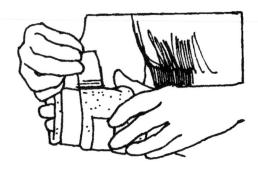

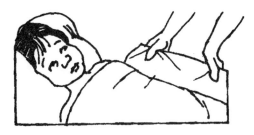

6 Keep the child warm and comforted.

7 Visit your local hospital emergency department or call your doctor as needed.

PREVENTION:

• Cover all electrical outlets.

• Keep electrical appliances away from water.

• Do not run extension cords under carpets.

Burns: Heat/Flames

PROTECT YOURSELF. DO NOT PROCEED INTO AN ENCLOSED AREA OR BURNING HOUSE. BE SURE IT IS SAFE.

MAY SEE:

First-Degree Burns
- minor burn
- skin is red and sensitive (like sunburn)

Second-Degree Burns
- skin red, blistered, swollen
- very painful (like peeling with sunburn)

Third-Degree Burns
- white or blackened
- may be leathery
- no pain at burn but painful at edges

 Stop the burning process. If flames are present, roll the child on the ground, smother flames with a blanket or soak with water.

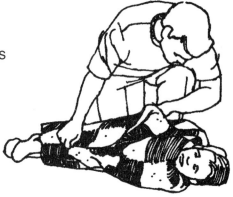

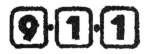 Call 9-1-1 or your local Emergency Medical Services number if any of the following are present:
- burns are severe or on the face
- there is a lot of smoke in the room
- the child is under two years of age
- not breathing or unconscious refer to:

BREATHING/C.P.R.		UNCONSCIOUS	
0 to 1 year	Page 34	0 to 1 year	Page 172
Over 1 year	Page 38	Over 1 year	Page 176

 Remove loose clothes from the burn area and remove all jewelery. Do not attempt to remove any burned-on fabric.

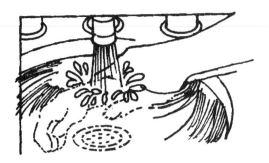

 Soak the burn area with room temperature water for five minutes.

 Wrap the child in clean, dry blankets or sheets.

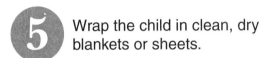

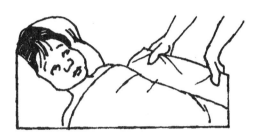

 Visit your local hospital emergency department or call your doctor.

COMMENTS:

• Never use butter, lotions or ointments on burns unless prescribed.

PREVENTION:

• Keep lighters/matches out of reach of children.

• Keep flammables in a locked cupboard.

• When running a bath, turn cold water **ON** first and hot water **OFF** first.

• Keep kettles empty of hot fluids.

• Keep pot handles turned toward the back of the stove.

• Always supervise small children in the kitchen and in bathrooms.

• Keep the hot water heater temperature at a minimal temperature.

Carbon Monoxide Poisoning

MAY SEE:
- dizziness
- headaches
- pink to cherry red skin color
- confusion
- vomiting
- convulsions
- unconsciousness

 Take the child into fresh air.

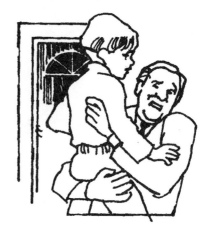

  Call 9-1-1 or your local Emergency Medical Services number.

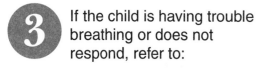 If the child is having trouble breathing or does not respond, refer to:

BREATHING/C.P.R.	
0 to 1 year	Page 34
Over 1 year	Page 38

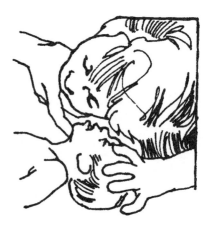

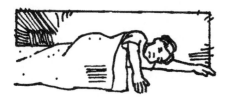 Keep the child warm and safe until help arrives.

COMMENTS:

You are also at risk from the gas. Do not stay in the area for long periods of time when you are attempting to remove the child.

PREVENTION:

- Do not leave children alone in running cars.

- Install a carbon monoxide sensor in your home.

- Clean and repair chimneys and gas vents at least yearly.

- Have natural gas appliances inspected at least annually by licensed gas contractors. Some companies offer this service free of charge.

NOTES:

Chest Pain

 Call 9-1-1 or your local Emergency Medical Services number if chest pain is accompanied by:
- injury to the chest
- shortness of breath
- increased pain with a deep breath
- high fever
- coughing up blood
- other signs of serious illness

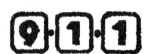

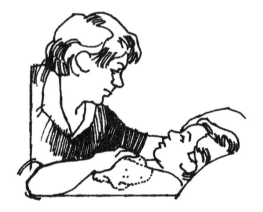

 Mild chest pain may be eased by applying warmth.

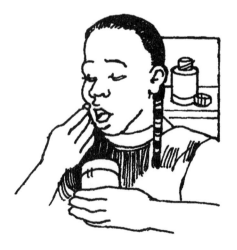 The child may use medication for pain (e.g., acetaminophen - Tylenol or Tempra), as directed by your doctor.

A harsh cough may cause chest soreness. Check with your doctor about the cause of the cough.

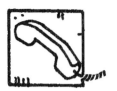

 Call your doctor or visit your local hospital emergency department as needed.

NOTES:

Chicken Pox

MAY SEE:
- small red bumps
- headache
- sores with white or clear or yellow centers
- itching, crusting
- fever

NOTE: Chicken pox often begin on back and chest and may spread.

 Apply calamine lotion to the welts to relieve itch.

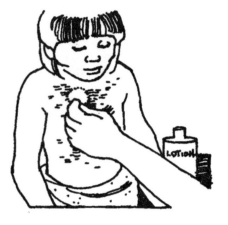

 If fever is present, see **Fever** on page 98.

Lukewarm baths with baking soda or a commercial oatmeal bath product may also help to relieve itch.

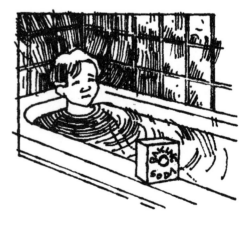

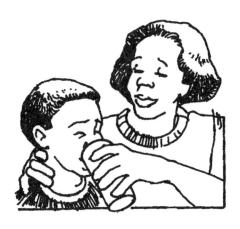

 4 Encourage the child to drink fluids, especially if he or she is feverish.

 5 Cut the child's fingernails short to help prevent infection from scratching. If itching is not relieved by the calamine lotion, consult your doctor for an alternate treatment.

COMMENTS:

- Chicken Pox has a three-week incubation period and is contagious five days before the rash starts and until the pox starts to dry.

- Avoid contact with children outside the home during this time. Notify your child's school, day care or babysitter and keep the child at home.

- Do not give A.S.A. (Aspirin) as it puts your child at risk for Reyes Syndrome, an illness which can harm the liver and brain.

Choking And Conscious *(Newborn To 1 Year)*

MAY SEE: • cough • pink color

Stay with the infant and encourage him or her to cough.

MORE SERIOUS SYMPTOMS MAY BE:

- becoming limp
- unable to cough/cry/speak
- paleness/blue in color
- very, very rapid breathing
- making high-pitched grunting or wheezing noises with breathing
- nostrils flaring; infant seems to be working very hard to breath
- infant seems to be unable to recognize parents or loved ones
- skin on chest and/or throat seems to be "sucking in" with breathing
- infant needs to sit up to breathe or has difficulty breathing while lying down

NOTE: Any child or infant having trouble breathing or struggling to breath should not be given food or drink until so advised by medical personnel.

 DO NOT LEAVE THE INFANT. If possible, have someone else call 9-1-1 or your local Emergency Medical Services number, or take the infant with you and call now.

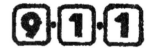

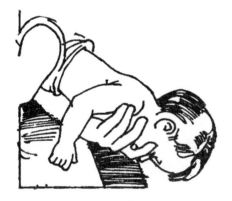

 Support the infant by holding the head with one hand, cupping the jaw and resting the body on your forearms.

Lower the head, supporting the infant on your lap. Try to keep the head down.

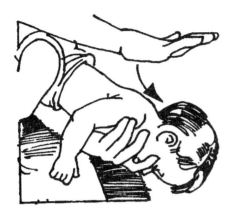

 Give up to 5 back blows between the shoulder blades, using the heel of your hand.

5 Turn over and give up to five chest thrusts one finger width below the nipple line, over the breast bone. Press chest down approximately half to one inch each time.

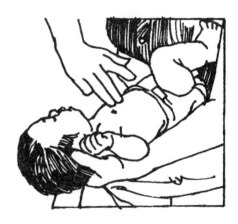

6 Repeat back blows and chest thrusts until effective or infant becomes unconscious (looks like he or she is asleep). (NOTE: always try to keep the head down.)

Refer to:

CHOKING & UNCONSCIOUS	
0 to 1 year	Page 58
Over 1 year	Page 60

Choking And Unconscious (Newborn To 1 Year)

MAY SEE:
- was awake and choking but is now unresponsive
- not crying, speaking or coughing
- pale or blue in color
- looks asleep (unconscious)

 If you are not alone, have someone call 9-1-1 or your local Emergency Medical Services number.

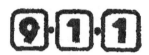

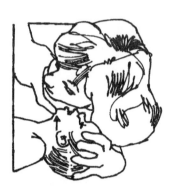

② AIRWAY A

Grab the chin and tongue with one hand and pull forward "Tongue/Jaw Lift". Look in the mouth. ONLY if you see an object in the mouth, gently sweep the mouth with two fingers to remove the object.

If you suspect a neck injury due to a fall or a motor vehicle accident, etc., carefully perform the chin lift to avoid twisting the neck.

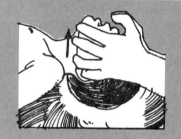

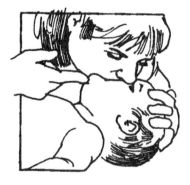

③ BREATHING B

Try to breathe for the infant covering the mouth and nose with your mouth.

④ If the airway is still blocked, reposition head and try to breathe for the infant again.

5 If airway is still blocked give up to five back blows between the shoulder blades, using the heel of your hand. Follow by up to five chest thrusts.

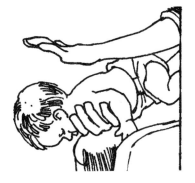

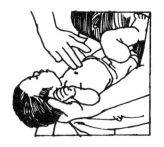

6 Repeat steps two to five until effective or until approximately one minute has gone by.

7 If no one has called 9-1-1 or your local Emergency Medical Services number, take the infant with you to the phone and call now.

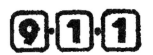

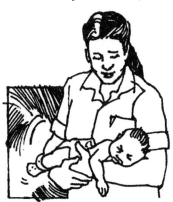

8 If the infant starts to breathe on his or her own, place the infant on one side. Avoid placing an infant on his or her side if you suspect a neck injury. This should be done by trained medical personnel. See **Back And Neck Injury** on page 20.

9 If air enters the airway but the infant is still unconscious (sleeping), perform rescue breathing at a rate of one breath every three seconds or 20 breaths per minute.

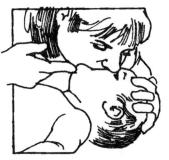

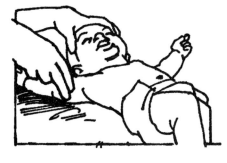

10 CIRCULATION **C**
Check pulse - if no pulse start C.P.R.:

BREATHING/C.P.R.	
0 to 1 year	Page 34
Over 1 year	Page 38

Choking And Conscious *(Children Over 1 Year)*

MAY SEE: • good cough   • pink color

Stay with the child and encourage him or her to cough.

MORE SERIOUS SYMPTOMS MAY BE:

- becoming limp
- paleness/blue in color
- unable to cough/cry/speak
- very, very rapid breathing
- making high-pitched grunting or wheezing noises with breathing
- nostrils flaring; child seems to be working very hard to breath
- child seems to be unable to recognize parents or loved ones
- skin on chest and/or throat seems to be "sucking in" with breathing
- child needs to sit up to breathe or has difficulty breathing while lying down

NOTE: Any child or infant having trouble breathing or struggling to breath should not be given food or drink until so advised by medical personnel.

 DO NOT LEAVE THE CHILD. If possible, have someone else call 9-1-1 or your local Emergency Medical Services number.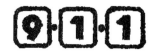

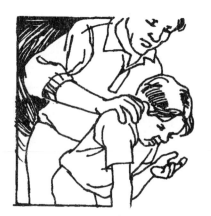

Encourage the child to cough. Ask "Are you choking?" "Can you talk?"

3 If the child is unable to speak/talk or has any of the above problems, give abdominal thrusts. Stand behind the child and place the flat part of your fist just above the belly button. Thrust inward and upward (like the letter "J").

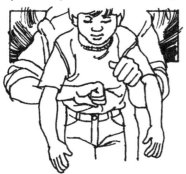 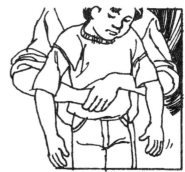

4 Repeat abdominal thrusts until effective OR child becomes unconscious (sleeping). See:

CHOKING & UNCONSCIOUS	
0 to 1 year	Page 58
Over 1 year	Page 60

PREVENTION:

An ounce of prevention is worth a pound of cure

- Cut food into small pieces and make sure infants or children chew food well.
- Popcorn, nuts, small candies should not be given to infants or children.
- Foods such as grapes, spaghetti, wieners, etc. should be cut into small chewable pieces.
- Infants or children should sit down to eat, never allow them to run around while eating.
- Always place infants or children in a car seat in the rear seat while riding in vehicles.
- Make sure all toys have secure pieces (e.g., eyes of stuffed animals won't pull off).
- Infants or children should wear helmets while in bicycle carriers or trailers.
- Cover electrical outlets.
- Keep children away from workshop areas.
- Keep matches out of infants' or children's reach.
- Make sure all medications and/or poisons are in a safe locked place.
- Keep balloons and rubber gloves away from infants or children.
- Keep drapery strings and any cords out of infants' or children's reach.
- Do not dress infants or children in clothing with a drawstring, hood or scarf when they may be playing on play structures.
- Make sure toilet seats are down.
- Keep small, shiny objects out of infants' or children's reach (e.g., coins, earrings, marbles).

Choking And Unconscious *(Child Over 1 Year)*

MAY SEE:
- was awake and choking but is now unresponsive
- not crying, speaking or coughing
- limp
- pale or blue in color
- looks asleep (unconscious)

 If possible, have someone else call 9-1-1 or your local Emergency Medical Services number.

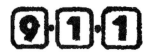

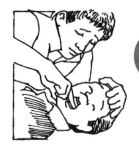

 AIRWAY

Grab the chin and tongue with one hand and pull forward "Tongue/Jaw Lift". Look in the mouth. ONLY if you see an object in the mouth, gently sweep the mouth with two fingers to remove the object.

If you suspect a neck injury due to a fall or a motor vehicle accident, etc., carefully perform the chin lift to avoid twisting the neck.

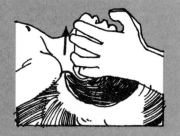

 BREATHING

Try to breathe for the child. If the child is small, you may need to cover the nose and mouth with your mouth.

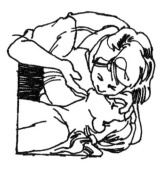

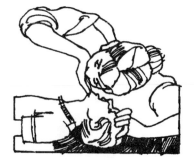

 If the airway is still blocked, reposition the head and try to breathe for the child again.

5 If the airway is still blocked, give up to five abdominal thrusts by straddling the child's legs and placing the heel of one hand just above the belly button. Push inwards and upwards. Do not sit on the child.

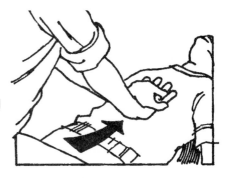

6 Repeat steps two to five until effective or until approximately one minute has gone by. If you are alone and the airway remains blocked, take the child with you to the phone and call 9-1-1 or your local Emergency Medical Services number.

7 If the child starts to breath on his or her own, place the child on one side. Avoid placing a child on his or her side if you suspect a neck injury. This should be done by trained medical personnel. **See Back And Neck Injury** on page 20.

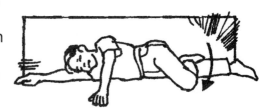

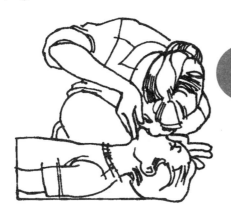

8 If air enters the airway but the child is still unconscious (sleeping), perform rescue breathing at a rate of one breath every three seconds or 20 breaths per minute.

9 Check pulse - if no pulse, start C.P.R. See:

BREATHING/C.P.R.	
0 to 1 year	Page 34
Over 1 year	Page 38

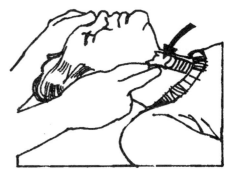

Colic

MAY SEE:
- loud crying
- irritability
- starts at one to four weeks of age
- most common in infants under three months of age
- draws legs up to abdomen
- sleeping during the day; but crying long and hard at night
- crying for long periods, and yet not sick or hungry
- content between crying spells
- feeds well and weight increasing

1 Call your doctor if the crying lasts more than three hours.

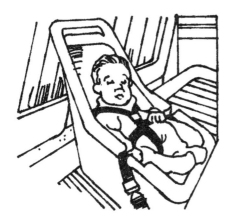

2 Movement, like walking, car rides, baby swings or a stroller may help. NEVER SHAKE AN INFANT.

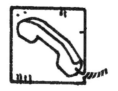

3 The following may help:
- cuddle, coo and rock the infant to make him or her feel secure
- hold the infant frequently and use a baby pouch like a "Snugly"
- try a soother
- smaller, frequent feedings; burp before, during and after
- wrap the infant snugly in a soft, stretchy blanket
- try to relax, infants can feel your tension.
- gentle massage
- the "colic carry" may be comforting (see diagram)
- music
- dim lights
- quiet room

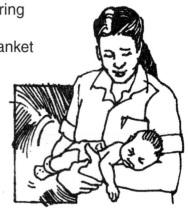

Avoid exposing infants to second-hand smoke.

 Get help and support from family, friends, a public health nurse or your doctor.

COMMENTS:

- The exact cause of colic is unknown, however it may be caused by:
  - too rapid feeding
  - over feeding
  - improper feeding, positioning and burping
  - overeating
  - swallowing too much air
  - illness
  - second-hand smoke

- If problems start after four weeks of age, there may be a physical or diet problem.

- If you are breast feeding, discuss your own diet with your doctor, public health nurse or lactation consultant.

- Do not change your infant's formula without consulting your doctor or a public health nurse.

Concussion *(See Also Head Injuries On Page 104))*

An injury to the head causing unconsciousness which may last from a few seconds to much longer. It may be mild or serious.

MAY SEE:
- confusion
- memory loss
- vomiting
- headache
- fatigue

 Call 9-1-1 or your local Emergency Medical Services number or visit your local hospital emergency department.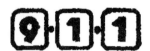

 If breathing stops, begin C.P.R. See:

BREATHING/C.P.R.	
0 to 1 year	Page 34
Over 1 year	Page 38

 If you suspect a back or neck injury, keep the child's head and body still. See **Back and Neck Injury** on Page 20.

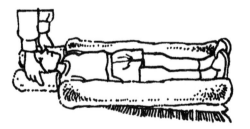

 If bleeding is present, apply light pressure with a clean cloth or towel. See **Cuts** on Page 74.

5 Do not give the child food or drink.

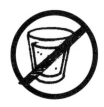

COMMENTS:

A child with a mild concussion may not need to be admitted to hospital. The doctor in the emergency department will decide if he or she can go home. If the child develops any of the following problems, bring him or her back to the hospital immediately:

- abnormal behaviour, drowsiness, irritability
- repeated vomiting
- slurred speech
- fever
- bleeding or clear fluid from nose or ears
- unable to wake them up
- severe headache
- seizures/convulsions
- blurry vision
- weakness in arms or legs
- uneven, dilated pupils (eyes)

Constipation

MAY SEE:
- abdominal pain
- lack of stools for longer period than usual for child
- soiling in underwear (older child)
- dry hard stools
- blood in stools
- leaking small amounts of liquid (infant)

 If the child is unable to pass stools for a long period, with continuous pain and discomfort or blood in stools, call your doctor.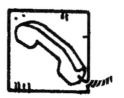

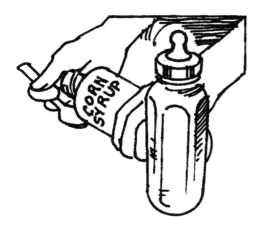

 Babies: Add 5 mL (1 teaspoon) of sugar or corn syrup to one 240 mL (8-ounce) bottle (use rarely).

Over 4 months: strained apricots, peaches, pears, prunes, diluted prune juice may help.

Children: Increase fruit and vegetables (e.g., prunes, figs, raisins, beans, celery and lettuce, bran cereals and muffins, crackers, prune juice).

Avoid enemas, suppositories or laxatives, unless recommended by your doctor.

COMMENTS:
- Babies, especially breast-fed babies, may normally have very infrequent stools. Watch for other signs of discomfort.
- Adding sugar to bottles should not be done regularly. Do this only to treat occasional constipation. If you need to use this more frequently, see your doctor.
- Constipation may be caused by certain foods, sickness, change in environment (e.g., afraid to use the school's toilet).

PREVENTION:
- Eat a well-balanced diet with plenty of fruit and vegetables. Prepare baby formula exactly as directed, formula that is too strong or too weak may cause serious health problems.
- Know your child's bowel habits.

NOTES:

Convulsions/Seizures/Fits

MAY SEE:
- jerking of arms, legs or head
- fluttering of eyes or drooling
- blue around lips

 If the child is not breathing or responding, call 9-1-1 or your local Emergency Medical Services number. Refer to:

9·1·1

BREATHING/C.P.R.		UNCONSCIOUS	
0 to 1 year	Page 34	0 to 1 year	Page 172
Over 1 year	Page 38	Over 1 year	Page 176

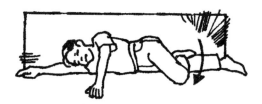

2 If the child is breathing, turn the child onto one side to prevent him or her from choking.

3 Keep the child safe and free from injury. Move any objects which may cause injury.

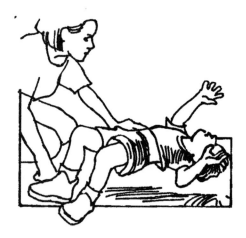

4 Do not put anything into the child's mouth.

Do not try to hold the child still.

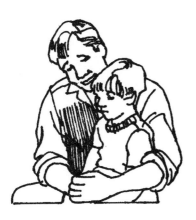

 When the convulsion stops, reassure the child and be calm. The child may be confused for a while and may not be able to understand you.

 Visit your local hospital emergency department or call your doctor.

COMMENTS:

- A seizure may be caused by:

    - infection
    - **Fever** (especially in the first 12 to 24 hours of the fever), see page 98
    - **Head Injuries**, see page 104
    - serious illness

- Do not give the child anything to eat or drink until he or she is fully awake and alert.

- A seizure will usually not cause permanent injury.

Croup

MAY SEE:
- a barky, harsh cough
- hoarse voice
- noisy breathing
- difficulty swallowing
- skin on chest, neck or throat seems to be "sucking in" with breathing
- sore throat
- fever and restlessness

 If the child has difficulty breathing call 9-1-1 or your local Emergency Medical Services number. Refer to:

BREATHING/C.P.R.	
0 to 1 year	Page 34
Over 1 year	Page 38

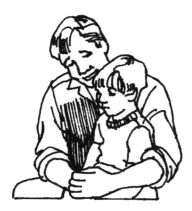

2 If the child has a harsh, barking cough with noisy breathing keep him or her in a comfortable sitting position.

3 Provide cool humidity (e.g., humidifier, a shower, or cool outside air).

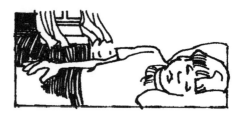

 4 If the child does not improve, visit your local hospital emergency department.

5 If the child has a **Fever,** see page 98.

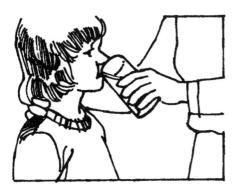

6 Have the child drink lots of clear fluids.

COMMENTS:
- Like a cold virus, the virus that causes croup is spread through the air when coughing or sneezing.
- Croup usually occurs in children aged 3 months to 4 years.

Cuts

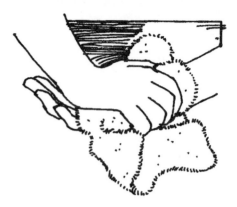

1 Apply direct pressure to the cut with your hand or a clean cloth or towel.

2 If bleeding is severe, call 9-1-1 or call your local Emergency Medical Services number.

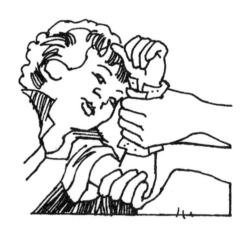

3 Elevate the limb above the heart, unless you suspect a broken bone. See **Broken Bones** on page 40.

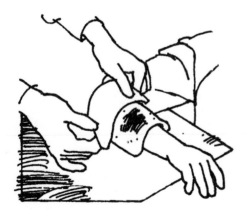

4 If the cloth or towel becomes soaked with blood, DO NOT REMOVE IT. Place another clean cloth/towel on top with direct pressure (repeat this step as necessary).

Visit your local hospital emergency department or call your doctor, for advice as to whether or not stitches are needed.

COMMENTS:

After the bleeding stops, clean the cut with water and use clean bandages to cover the cut. Check the limb frequently for new bleeding. If the limb is cold or blue, the bandage is likely too tight.

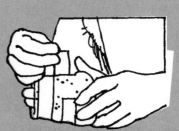

PREVENTION:

• Ensure your child is fully immunized to prevent Tetanus/Lockjaw.

• Supervise your child. Keep dangerous or sharp objects out of reach.

• Child proof your home.

Dehydration

MAY SEE:

Mild
- dry mouth
- fewer tears
- urinates (pees) slightly or in smaller amounts

Moderate
(mild signs plus)
- dry skin
- sunken eyes
- sunken soft spot (fontanelle) on head
- irritable
- listlessness
- no tears

Severe
(mild and moderate signs plus)
- weight loss
- cool, pale skin
- weakness
- unconsciousness
- no urination
- rapid breathing
- weak pulse

NOTE: SEVERE DEHYDRATION IS A LIFE-THREATENING CONDITION

 If dehydration is severe, call 9-1-1 or your local Emergency Medical Services number.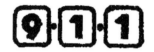

  If dehydration is moderate, call your doctor or visit your local hospital emergency department.

If dehydration is mild:
- encourage the child to drink frequent small amounts of water, fruit juices or flat soft drinks such as ginger ale
- if the child cannot drink, offer chips of ice, frozen juices or popsicles
- if **Vomiting,** see page 182
- if **Diarrhea** is present, see page 78

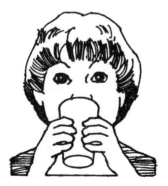 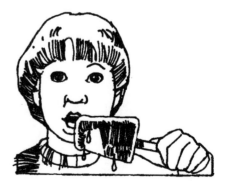

COMMENTS:

- Obtain medical assistance as required, to keep the proper amount of fluids and nutrients in the body to prevent dehydration.

- Discuss using over-the-counter medications (e.g., Gravol) with your doctor or pharmacist.

PREVENTION:

- Have the child drink plenty of fluids.

NOTES:

Diarrhea

• frequent, watery stools
(bowel movement)
• stools that are an unusual color

• foul-smelling stools
• blood in stools

 If diarrhea occurs more than once each hour and lasts for more than 12 hours, or there is accompanying fever, stomach ache, or blood in the diarrhea, call your doctor.

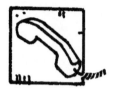

 If the child has a dry mouth, sunken eyes, fever, decreased urine output, and is listless, or is difficult to waken, call your doctor or visit your local hospital emergency department immediately.

Offer small amounts of clear fluids such as water, flat ginger ale, or a commercially prepared electrolyte replacement (e.g., Pedialyte, Gastrolyte).

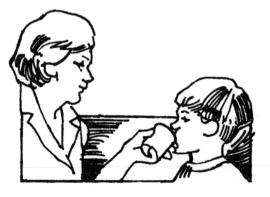

It may be helpful to avoid milk products or hard-to-digest foods for a few days.

 Use a diaper cream to protect the child's bottom from irritation.

COMMENTS:

Diarrhea can be caused by viruses, bacteria, parasites, poor diet, some medications and an allergy to milk or food.

Breast-fed infants' stools are often loose and frequent. Know your child's bowel habits.

PREVENTION:

- Sterilize baby formula equipment and bottles for young infants.
- Discard unused formula after each feeding; do not offer old formula.
- Wash your hands after going to the bathroom or changing a diaper and before preparing food.
- Eat a well-balanced diet.
- Cook foods completely.
- Keep hot foods hot and cold foods cold.

Dislocated Joints *(Elbow/Shoulder)*

MAY SEE:
- pain
- unusual shape of joint
- tingling
- bluish color

- swelling
- not using limb
- numbness

 Do not move the child, unless he or she is in further danger, until the limb is immobilized.

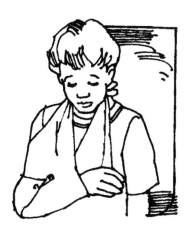

 Immobilize the limb, see **Broken Bones** on page 40.

 Depending on the severity of the situation, call 9-1-1 or your local Emergency Medical Services number or call your doctor or visit your local hospital emergency department.

PREVENTION:

- Supervise children at play.
- Never yank or pull a child by the arm.
- Don't swing or lift a child by the arms.

NOTES:

Drooling/Epiglottitis

Epiglottitis: Difficulty swallowing, sore throat, drooling

MAY SEE:
- high fever
- difficulty breathing, especially when lying down
- bluish color of lips and skin
- frightened, anxious
- no cough
- looks very ill
- sits forward and does not want to change position

- severe sore throat
- croaking sound with breathing
- fussy, restless
- drooling, difficulty swallowing
- muffled voice
- usually comes on suddenly and gets worse quickly

 Call 9-1-1 or your local Emergency Medical Services number immediately or take the child directly to your local hospital emergency department.

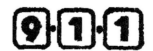

 If child stops breathing, refer to:

BREATHING/C.P.R.	
0 to 1 year	Page 34
Over 1 year	Page 38

 Do not irritate or disturb the child (e.g., do not take the child's temperature).

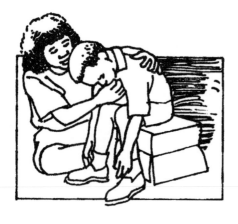

Do not attempt to change the child's position. The most comfortable position is usually sitting up and leaning forward (often best on the parent's lap).

Do not attempt to look into the child's mouth or throat.

  Do not give the child anything to eat or drink.

 Apply cold mist or cold air (e.g., humidifier, a shower, or cool outside air) to the child until emergency help arrives (ONLY IF IT DOES NOT UPSET THE CHILD).

 When emergency help arrives, the child may best be transported sitting on the parent's lap to avoid further upset.

COMMENT:
• The drooling and sore throat that occurs with Epiglottitis is more severe than baby drooling that is caused by teething. It is a true medical emergency.

PREVENTION:
• Keep children fully immunized.

Drowning: Water

1 Remove the child from the water. Be sure to support the child's head and neck, keeping them level and in line with the rest of the body.

2 If the child is not breathing, begin C.P.R, See:

BREATHING/C.P.R.	
0 to 1 year	Page 34
Over 1 year	Page 38

Have another person call 9-1-1 or your local Emergency Medical Services number.

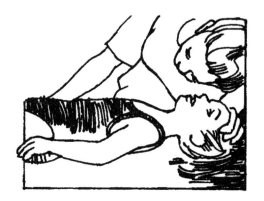

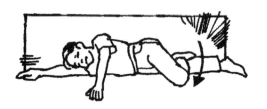

3 If the child is breathing but unconscious, lay him or her on one side. See:

UNCONSCIOUS	
0 to 1 year	Page 172
Over 1 year	Page 176

If the child vomits, keep him or her on one side and clean out the mouth.

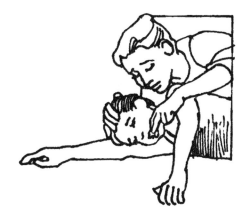

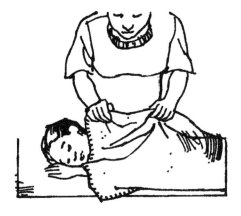

 Keep the child warm. Do not try to get the child to eat or drink.

Call your doctor or visit your local hospital emergency department.

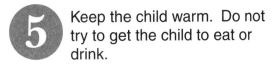

PREVENTION:

- Never leave small children alone in the bathtub, even for a few moments.
- Supervise children when they are playing near water.
- Life jackets (personal flotation devices) should be worn in a boat and when swimming.
- Pools should be surrounded by a high, locked fence.
- For small children, keep bathroom doors closed and toilet seats locked.
- Teach children to swim.
- Keep all containers with liquid closed (e.g., diaper pails, toilets, barrels, hot tubs).

Drowning: Suffocation

MANURE PITS:
- DO NOT ENTER A MANURE PIT UNDER ANY CIRCUMSTANCES without a self-contained breathing apparatus.
- Deadly gases that are heavier than air will kill very quickly.

LAGOONS:
- DO NOT ENTER, there may be a crust on top but it will not likely support your body weight.
- Deadly gases and poisons will kill you quickly.

GRANARY BINS OR WAGONS:
- DO NOT ENTER the space as you may become trapped too.
- Shut off all power sources and heating units to the space.

OTHER:
- DO NOT ENTER other like situations such as, deep wells or cisterns; unstable piles of snow, sand or earth.

 Call 9-1-1 or your local fire department and your local Emergency Medical Services number.

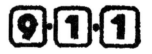

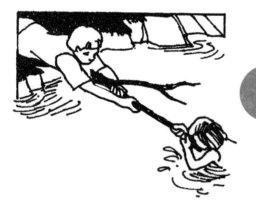

If the victim is conscious, throw a rope or other line to try and pull him or her out.

Once you get the child out, keep him or her warm. Do not try to get the child to eat or drink.

PREVENTION:

- Never leave children unsupervised near open pits, pools, lagoons or other structures in which they may become trapped.

- Educate children on local hazards and safety procedures.

NOTES:

Earache

MAY SEE:
- fever
- yellow or green ear drainage
- irritable, often while lying down
- difficulty hearing
- pain
- pulling at the ears
- redness
- diarrhea in children under two years

1 Call your doctor and have the child's ear examined.

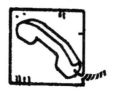

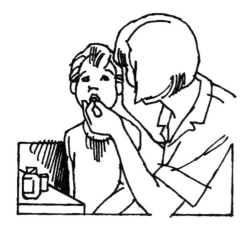

2 Give acetaminophen (e.g., Tylenol or Tempra) to ease discomfort and/or fever. See bottle for instructions.

3 Ice in a wash cloth on the ear, for 15 minutes, may also help the pain go away.

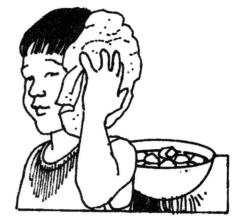

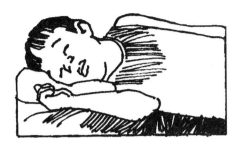

 Have the child lie on the same side as the ear that hurts. If the child is older than 12 months, elevate his or her head slightly on pillows.

 Do not put anything in the ear, such as water or oil, unless directed to do so by your doctor.

COMMENTS:

- An earache is usually caused by an infection in the inner, middle or outer ear canal or by an object or insect that is stuck in the ear.

- Most earaches will end in one to two days with acetaminophen

- If earache is associated with high fever, or reoccurs, see your doctor.

Ears: Foreign Objects

MAY SEE:
- ringing in the ears
- itchiness
- ear drainage
- pain
- a very bad smell
- crusting of external ear canal

 Do not remove an object in the ear, even if you can see it. You may push it in deeper, by mistake, or break the ear drum.

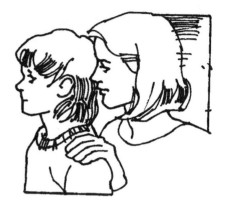

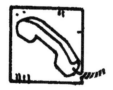 Call your doctor or visit your local hospital emergency department.

Discourage the child from poking at his or her ear.

90

COMMENTS:
• The foreign object may be a small insect.

PREVENTION:
• Keep small objects away from children under three years of age.
• Supervise children carefully. They frequently put small objects (e.g., food, small toys, stones) into any body opening.
• Teach children not to put small objects into any body openings.

NOTES:

Eyes: Foreign Objects

MAY SEE:
- tearing
- redness
- child feels something in the eye
- burning
- may see an actual object stuck in eye
- cannot open eye
- pain
- scratchy feeling
- constantly blinking

OBJECT VISIBLE AND STUCK IN EYE:

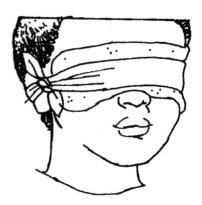

1 If the object is stuck into the eyeball, cover both eyes loosely with a bandage or scarf. DO NOT TRY TO REMOVE THE OBJECT.

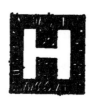

2 Contact your doctor immediately or go to your local hospital emergency department.

OBJECT NOT VISIBLE/NOT STUCK IN EYE:

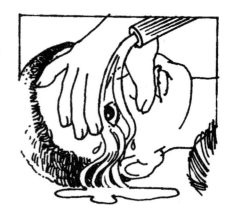

1 Hold the child's head under a gentle stream of clean, warm water or pour from a glass across the eye surface, with the affected eye down. Do this for a few minutes then recheck to see if object is gone.

2 Do not rub the child's eyes; encourage the child not to rub his or her eye.

3 If an object is visible in the lower eyelid try to remove it with the corner of a clean, moistened cloth.

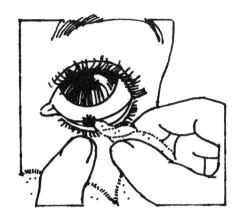

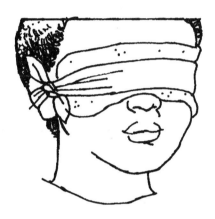

4 If you are unable to remove the object, cover both eyes loosely with a bandage or scarf and immediately call your doctor or visit the local hospital emergency department.

PREVENTION:
- Teach children to not put anything in their eyes.
- Keep children away from areas where there is flying debris.
- Adults must keep a close watch over young children at play.
- If "helping" with carpentry, etc., children should wear safety glasses as well.

Eye Infection

MAY SEE:
- redness of white part of eye
- watery or sticky drainage from eye (color may be yellow, green or brown)
- eyelids may stick together
- feel something in the eye (irritation, discomfort)
- eye may be puffy

 Encourage the child NOT TO RUB HIS OR HER EYES.

2 DO NOT SQUEEZE any swelling on the eyes or eyelids.

3 If there is any eye drainage or discharge, gently wipe the eye, from the center outwards, with a clean, damp cloth. Use a different part of the washcloth for each eye.

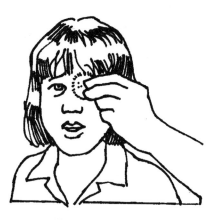

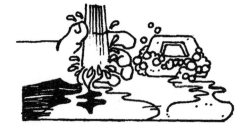

 The caregiver and the child should wash their hands carefully after touching the child's eye and after eye care.

 Keep the child's face cloth and towels separate from the other children's.

6 Call your doctor if the infection persists or if you are concerned.

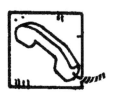

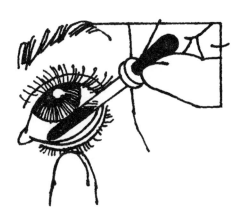

7 After the eye is washed, apply eye medication as directed by your doctor.

COMMENTS:
- Eye infections spread easily from one child to another.
- Your child's school or day care should be informed.

PREVENTION:
- Teach children to not put things in their eyes.
- Teach children to properly wash their hands and encourage them to do it frequently.

Fainting

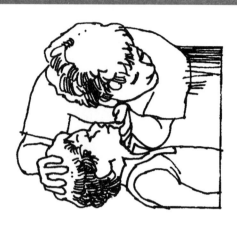

1 Check for breathing. If the child is not breathing, refer to:

BREATHING/C.P.R.	
0 to 1 year	Page 34
Over 1 year	Page 38

2 If the child is unconscious, see:

UNCONSCIOUS	
0 to 1 year	Page 172
Over 1 year	Page 176

3 Lay the child flat; loosen the collar.

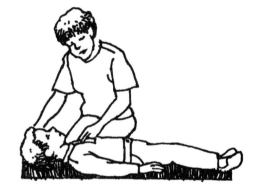

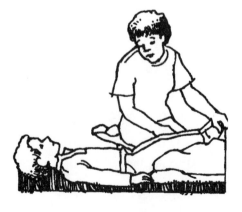

4 Raise the child's legs above the level of the head.

5 Provide cool cloths for the child's face and neck.

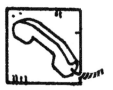

6 Call your doctor if there is no obvious reason for the fainting.

COMMENTS:
- Fainting may be caused by:
  - drug or chemical misuse or abuse
  - a bump to the head or a head injury
  - low blood sugar
  - **Fever** (see page 98) or **Heat Exhaustion** (see page 110)
  - serious illness
  - overreaction or excitement

Fever

- fast breathing
- tiredness
- sweating
- loss of appetite
- skin warm to touch
- pale or flushed appearance
- chills
- glossy eyes
- fussiness
- high temperature

1 Call your doctor or visit your local hospital emergency department if:
- fever persists for 24 hours for no obvious reason (e.g., flu, chicken pox)
- fever in an infant under six months
- for children over six months, if fever persists longer than 24 hours
- a high fever which can not be reduced within four to six hours
- fever is accompanied by other signs of serious illness such as stiff neck, **Dehydration** (see page76), severe vomiting, confusion
- **Convulsions** occur (see page70)

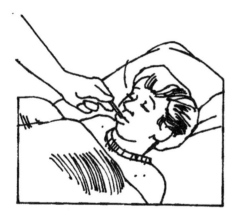

2 Check temperature every four hours until the fever ends.
- The average oral temperature range is 36.5 to 37.5° C (97.7 to 99.5° F)
- The average armpit temperature range is 36.0 to 37.0° C (96.8 to 98.6° F)

3 Make the child more comfortable: dress in cool, cotton clothing; sponge with lukewarm water. Stop sponging if child starts shivering.

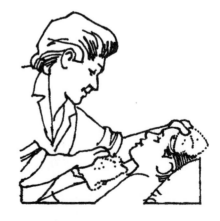

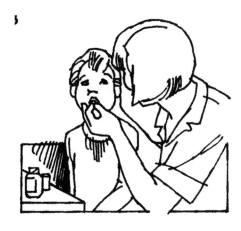

 Give the child acetaminophen (e.g., Tylenol or Tempra) as directed on the bottle or by your doctor.

 Encourage the child to drink plenty of fluids. You may try popsicles, freezies or ginger ale.

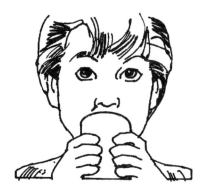

COMMENTS:
- Do not give A.S.A. (Aspirin) as it puts your child at risk for Reyes Syndrome, an illness which can harm the liver and brain.
- If you are unsure of how to take your child's temperature, contact your public health nurse or doctor.

Frostbite

MAY SEE:
- white, waxy and hard skin
- numbness or loss of feeling in frostbitten area
- bluish-white skin (deep frostbite)
- blisters
- pain or stinging in the frostbitten area

 Remove any tight objects such as rings, bracelets, gloves or boots.

 Do not rub the frostbitten area, handle gently.

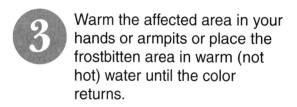 Warm the affected area in your hands or armpits or place the frostbitten area in warm (not hot) water until the color returns.

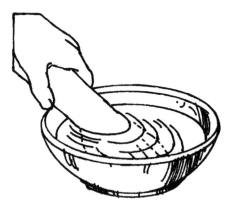

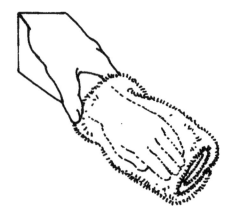

 Do not break blisters. Cover the frostbitten area with a loose, dry, clean cloth or dressing.

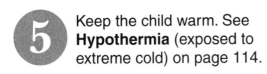

5 Keep the child warm. See **Hypothermia** (exposed to extreme cold) on page 114.

6 Do not allow the child to walk if his or her feet are affected.

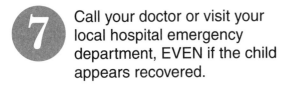

7 Call your doctor or visit your local hospital emergency department, EVEN if the child appears recovered.

Frostbite

COMMENTS:
- Ensure that children wear appropriate head, hand and foot wear.
- Layer clothing for warmth.
- Be aware of your local weather conditions. Limit children's outdoor activities during severe weather conditions, extreme cold and high wind chill.

Headache

MAY SEE: Complaints of pain anywhere within the head, including the eyes.

 Contact your doctor if the headache:
- repeatedly wakes your child up from sleep
- is accompanied by fever
- is severe and unrelieved
- is accompanied by vomiting
- is accompanied by neck or spine ache
- commonly occurs in the morning

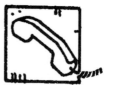

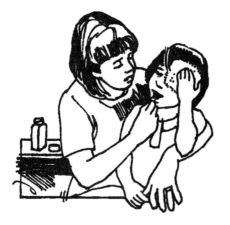

 Give acetaminophen (e.g., Tylenol or Tempra) as directed.

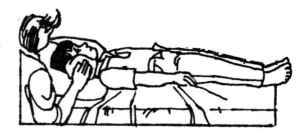

A cold cloth on the forehead or neck and rest in a dark room may help.

COMMENTS:

Headaches may be due to infection, head or neck injury, tension or stress, vision problems or disease.

NOTES:

Head Injuries (*Concussions*)

Mild
- headache
- brief loss of consciousness (not responding)
- confusion for a few seconds
- younger children should cry immediately
- older children should be able to answer simple questions
- vomiting may be present

Severe
- unconsciousness (not responding) lasting longer than a few seconds
- persistent drowsiness
- convulsions
- vomiting
- confusion
- clear or bloody fluid draining from nose or ears

 Call 9-1-1 or your local Emergency Medical Services number, or visit your local hospital emergency department.

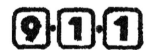

 If breathing stops, begin C.P.R., see:

BREATHING/C.P.R.		UNCONSCIOUS	
0 to 1 year	Page 34	0 to 1 year	Page 172
Over 1 year	Page 38	Over 1 year	Page 176

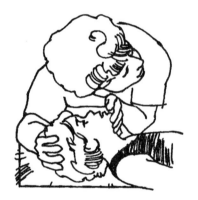

 If you suspect a back or neck injury DO NOT MOVE THE CHILD. Wait for medical help. See **Back And Neck Injury** on page 20.

 For a sports-related injury DO NOT REMOVE HELMET unless necessary for C.P.R.

If a cut or other wound is bleeding, apply light pressure with a clean cloth or gauze.

 If clear or bloody fluid is draining from nose or ears, do not attempt to stop the flow. Use a clean cloth or gauze to absorb the fluid.

 Do not give the child anything to eat or drink.

COMMENTS:

A child with a mild concussion may not need to be admitted to the hospital. The doctor in the emergency department of your local hospital will decide if the child can go home. If the child develops any of the following problems, bring him or her back to the hospital immediately:

- abnormal behavior
- repeated vomiting
- slurred speech
- drowsiness
- fever
- irritability
- weakness in arms or legs

- pupils of eyes are unequal in size
- unable to wake up the child
- severe headache
- seizures/convulsions
- blurry vision
- bleeding or clear fluid from nose or ears

Head Lice

MAY SEE: • Pearly, tear-drop-shaped eggs (nits) that are firmly attached to the hair, within a couple of inches of the scalp.

 Do not send children to school or day care until treated.

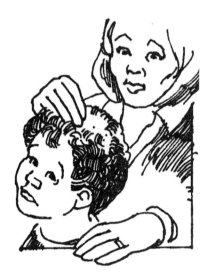

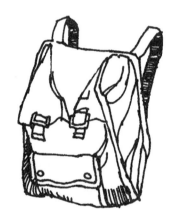 Check with your public health nurse, school nurse or doctor if you are unsure your family has head lice.

Notify the school or day care. They will send clothes home for cleaning, and will clean toys and make sure others do not have head lice.

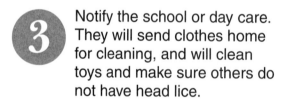

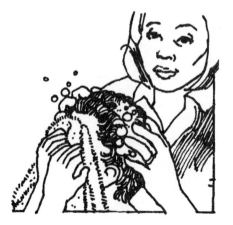

Buy the shampoo suggested by your pharmacist, nurse or doctor. Pregnant or nursing women and children under two years old need special treatment.

5 Follow the package instructions carefully. Use your fingertips or a fine-toothed comb to pull off all the nits after treatment.

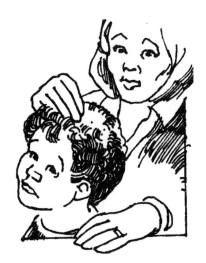

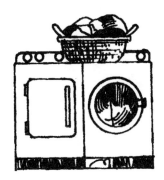

6 Wash all bedding, clothing and hair items. Vacuum your furniture and carpets.

7 Talk to your public health nurse for details about cleaning personal items.

8 Check other family members and follow the above steps.

PREVENTION:

- Get into the habit of checking family members weekly.

- Do not share combs or hats.

Heat Cramps

MAY SEE:
- muscle cramps
- nausea
- rapid heart rate
- weakness
- vomiting
- pale and sweating

 Move the child to a cool place and limit all activity.

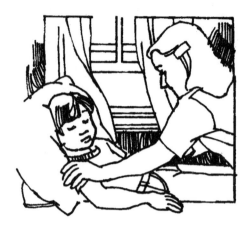

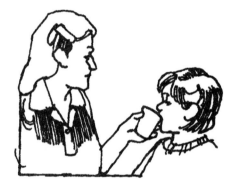

 Frequently, give the child small amounts of fruit juices or electrolyte drinks (e.g., Gatorade). Avoid soda pop and caffeine.

 If the child does not improve quickly, call your doctor or visit your local hospital emergency department.

PREVENTION:

- When the weather is very hot:
    - limit children's outdoor activities
    - provide fruit juice drinks frequently
    - watch for any changes in children's personality or physical condition
    - dress children according to the weather

- Salt tablets are not recommended for children.

- Never leave a child in a hot car, even for a short period of time.

- Provide children with an opportunity to cool down (e.g., lawn sprinklers).

- For rigorous physical activity:
    - bring a water bottle
    - drink a few ounces of water or a sports drink (e.g., Gatorade) whenever there is a break

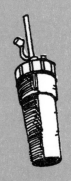

NOTES:

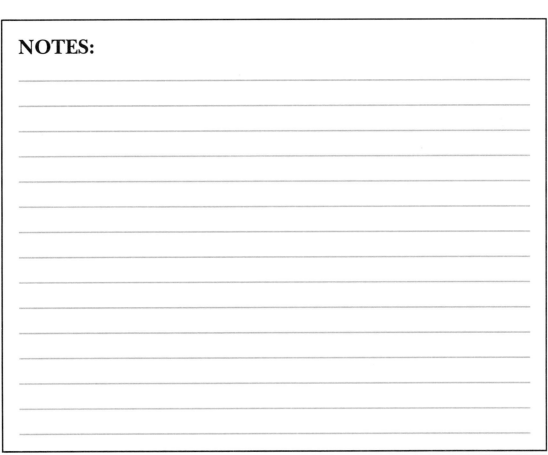

Heat Exhaustion

MAY SEE:
- muscle cramps
- nausea and vomiting
- thirst
- elevated temperature –
  38 to 40°C (100 to 104°F)
- weakness
- pale and sweating
- headache
- rapid heart rate

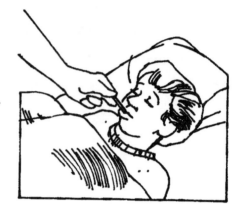

 If the child's temperature is greater than 40°C (104°F), refer to **Heat Stroke** on page 112.

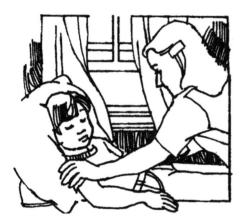

2 It is very important to quickly take the child to a cool place to rest.

3 Give the child fruit juices or electrolyte drinks (e.g., Gatorade).

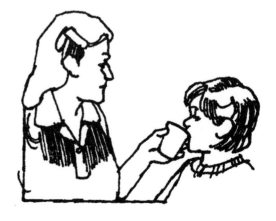

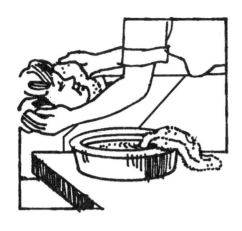

 4 If the child's temperature is elevated, apply cool cloths to the child's face, neck, armpits and groin area.

 5 Call your doctor or take the child to your local hospital emergency department.

PREVENTION:
- When the weather is very hot:
    - limit children's outdoor activities
    - provide fruit juice drinks frequently
    - watch for any changes in children's personality or physical condition
    - dress children according to the weather
- Salt tablets are not recommended for children.
- Never leave a child in a hot car, even for a short period of time.
- Provide children with the opportunity to cool down (e.g., lawn sprinklers).
- For rigorous physical activity:
    - bring a water bottle
    - drink a few ounces of water or sports drink (e.g., Gatorade) whenever there is a break.

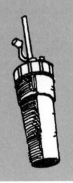

Heat Stroke

This a life threatening condition that may affect an active child in hot and/or humid weather.

MAY SEE:
- red, hot, dry skin
- restlessness and/or confusion
- convulsions
- elevated temperature – often over 40°C (104°F)

- dry mouth
- rapid heart rate
- unresponsiveness

Quickly move the child to a nearby cool place and call 9-1-1 or your local Emergency Medical Services number.

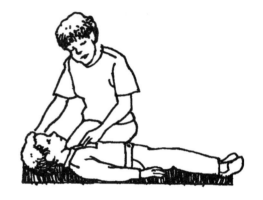

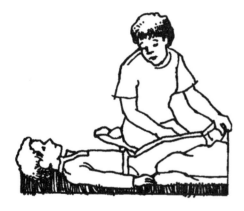

Remove the child's clothing and lay the child down in a cool place with feet elevated.

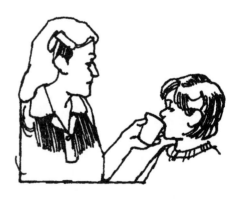

If awake and alert, give fruit juices or electrolyte drinks (e.g., Gatorade).

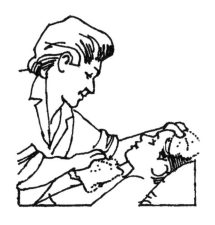

4 Reduce the child's temperature with cool cloths or covered ice packs applied to the child's face, neck, armpits and groin area.

5 Ensure the child is taken to your local hospital emergency department.

PREVENTION:
- When the weather is very hot:
    - limit children's outdoor activities
    - provide fruit juice drinks frequently
    - watch for any changes in children's personality or physical condition
    - dress children according to the weather
- Salt tablets are not recommended for children.
- Never leave a child in a hot car, even for a short period of time.
- Provide children with the opportunity to cool down (e.g., lawn sprinklers).
- For vigorous physical activity, bring a water bottle.
- Drink a few ounces every 10 to 20 minutes. Have a cup of water or sports drink (e.g., Gatorade) whenever there is a break.

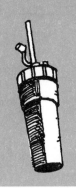

Hypothermia *(Extreme Cold)*

MAY SEE:
- shivering
- irritability
- drowsiness
- blurred vision

- child feels cold
- clumsiness
- slurred speech
- confused talk

The child may not notice these symptoms.

IN INFANTS:
- weak sucking
- bluish color to the face and limbs

- weak crying or no crying

AS HYPOTHERMIA INCREASES IN SEVERITY:
- shivering may stop
- unconsciousness

- stiff muscles

- In severe hypothermia the child may not respond, may not be breathing and may not have a pulse.

- Always obtain immediate emergency help; survival is possible even with prolonged exposure.

---

 1 Call 9-1-1 or your local Emergency Medical Services number. Refer to:

9·1·1

BREATHING/C.P.R.	
0 to 1 year	Page 34
Over 1 year	Page 38

UNCONSCIOUS	
0 to 1 year	Page 172
Over 1 year	Page 176

2 Carefully remove the child to a sheltered area.

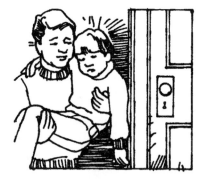

3 Gently remove any wet clothing.

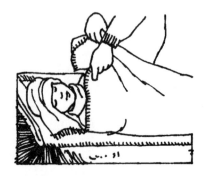

 4 Dress the child in dry clothes and cover with warm blankets. Cover head (except face) and neck.

Handle the child gently. Do not rub the skin. Keep the child still and quiet.

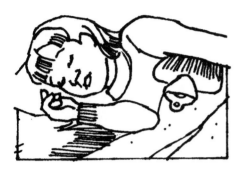

 Apply gentle heat to armpits and groin area with hot water bottles wrapped in towels.

 Do NOT give food or drink unless the child is alert.

8 Call your doctor or visit your local hospital emergency department, even if the child appears recovered.

COMMENT:
- If the child is fully awake and can swallow, give warm, sweet liquids (no alcohol).

PREVENTION:
- Store winter survival supplies in vehicles (emergency candles, blankets, food rations).
- Child-proof locks should be installed on residence doors to prevent chidren from wandering into severe weather.

Immunization Reaction

 After an immunization needle, give one dose of acetaminophen (e.g., Tylenol, Tempra) within the first hour (after measles, mumps and German measles needle, no medication will be needed immediately – reaction may be one to three weeks later).

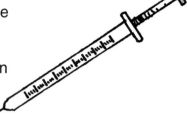

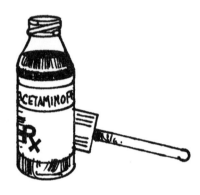

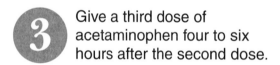 Give a second dose of acetaminophen four to six hours after the first dose.

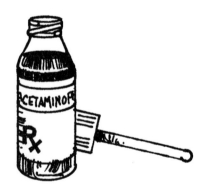

 Give a third dose of acetaminophen four to six hours after the second dose.

If your child has had febrile convulsions (seizures) in the past, give acetaminophen every four to six hours for 24 hours, see **Fever** on page 98.

Apply warm cloths or towels to the needle site for 15 minutes every hour, if the child's arm or leg is sore.

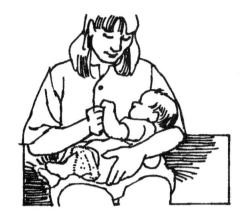

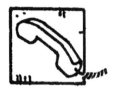

 If your child's fever does not subside, or if there are symptoms other than fever or mild discomfort, call your doctor.

COMMENT:
- Mild fever, irritability, and local tenderness are common immunization reactions.

Impaled Objects *(Stabbing, Nail, Fish Hook, Splinter)*

 DO NOT REMOVE the impaled object if it may cause further damage or increase bleeding.

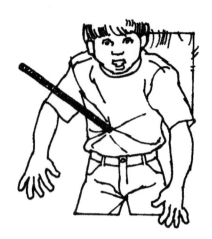

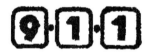 Call 9-1-1 or your local Emergency Medical Services number, if the child is having trouble breathing. See:

BREATHING/C.P.R.	
0 to 1 year	Page 34
Over 1 year	Page 38

3 If there is severe bleeding, call 9-1-1 or your local Emergency Medical Services number.

  Call your doctor or visit your local hospital emergency department for removal of the object.

If the object appears to be small enough to remove safely, sterile equipment should be used.

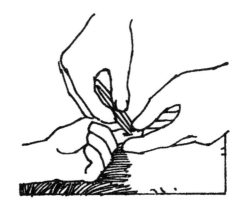

COMMENTS:
- Child may need immunization for Tetanus. Check your child's immunization record and ask your doctor.
- Watch for signs of infection following the removal of the impaled object (e.g., fever, redness and swelling, pain, drainage of pus).

Impetigo *(Skin Infection)*

MAY SEE:
- rash or sores that are crusty or have pus
- rash often around nose and/or mouth or may be anywhere

 Visit your doctor to get a prescription. Impetigo is easily treated with an antibacterial cream.

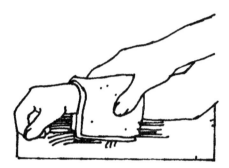

2 Soak the scabs or crusts off with warm water and a clean cloth.

3 Apply ointment as prescribed by your doctor.

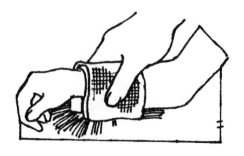

4 Keep sores loosely covered, unless they are on the child's face.

Discourage the child from scratching. Keep the child's fingernails short.

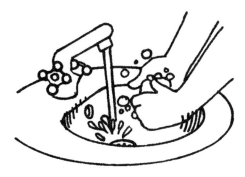

 Wash your hands and your child's hands often.

 Do not share toothbrushes or towels.

COMMENT:
- Children should stay home from school or day care until treatment has been started.

PREVENTION:
- Wash your hands and your child's hands often.
- Have children keep their hands away from their mouths and their noses.
- Do not share toothbrushes or towels.

Leg Pain

MAY SEE:
- redness
- lumps
- bruises
- fever
- reluctance to move the limb
- swelling
- warm areas
- bumps
- complaints of pain
- limping

 Try:
- rest
- cool compress
- mild pain relievers like acetaminophen (e.g., Tylenol or Tempra)
- elevate limb

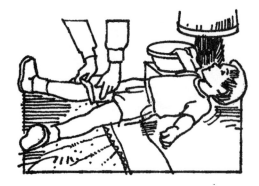

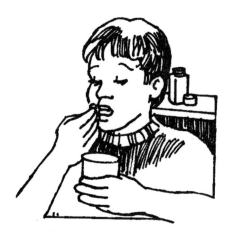

 Have your child examined by your doctor if the pain does not go away with the above treatments.

COMMENTS:

- Leg pains are often related to the normal growth of a child. But if it is a reoccuring pain in the same leg, see your doctor.

- Strenuous activity without sufficient warm up may cause leg pains.

NOTES:

Machinery Entanglement

1 Your safety comes first. Do not endanger yourself by entering an unsafe environment.

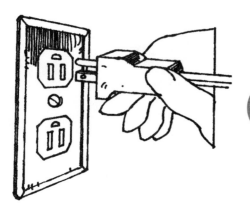

2 Turn off the machine's power source and stabilize any moving parts of the machinery.

3 Call 9-1-1 or your local Emergancy Medical Services number.

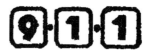

4 Check for breathing. If the child is not breathing, refer to:

BREATHING/C.P.R.	
0 to 1 year	Page 34
Over 1 year	Page 38

5 Check to see if the child is awake. If the child is not responsive, go to:

UNCONSCIOUS	
0 to 1 year	Page 172
Over 1 year	Page 176

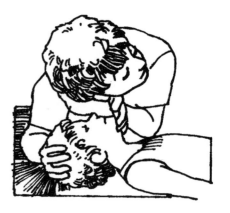

DO NOT REMOVE THE CHILD FROM THE MACHINE unless the child is in further danger, because you could cause further injury or death. Wait for your local rescue team to remove the child.

 Care for specific injuries as found. See the appropriate section in this book: **Unconscious** on page 172 (infants) or page 176 (children), **Cuts** on page 74, **Broken Bones** on page 40.

PREVENTION

- Ensure the child does not wear clothing that is too large, or has drawstrings, cords or hoods, around machinery.

- Ensure that all safety devices are working and in place.

- Long hair should be tied back when near machinery.

- Never leave a child unsupervised around machinery.

- Educate your children on local hazards and safety procedures.

Nose Bleed

MAY SEE:
- bleeding from the nose or mouth
- vomiting or spitting blood

 SEEK IMMEDIATE MEDICAL ATTENTION IF:
- bleeding cannot be controlled after 20 minutes of constant pressure
- the child was injured
- there are signs of serious illness present

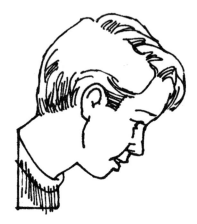

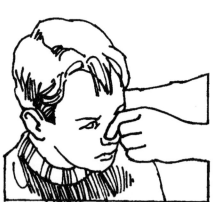

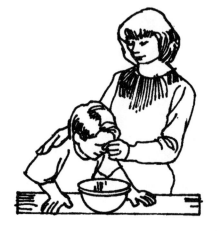

2 Sit the child down and tilt his or her head slightly forward.

3 Encourage slow, deep breathing through the mouth.

4 Pinch the child's nose firmly on the fleshy area just below the bony bridge area.

5 Maintain this position for **ten** minutes and have the child spit out any blood or fluid.

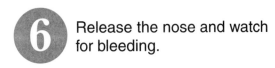

6 Release the nose and watch for bleeding.

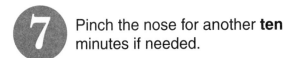

7 Pinch the nose for another **ten** minutes if needed.

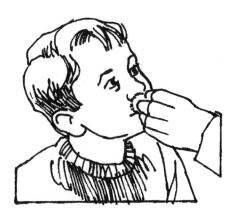

8 When the bleeding stops, clean the child's face with warm water.

9 The child should then rest quietly for at least 30 minutes (without blowing his or her nose).

COMMENTS:
- A child with a nose bleed should not lie down.
- Packing of the nose should not be attempted.
- See your doctor if your child has fequent nose bleeds.

PREVENTION
- Use a humidifier.
- Apply a thin layer of petroleum jelly to dry areas inside the nostrils.

Nose: Foreign Objects

MAY SEE:
- a very bad smell
- drainage from the nose
- you may actually see an object in the nose

 Unless the object can be easily removed and for small children who are unable to cooperate, it is safest to have the object removed by a doctor, as you may push it further in and cause more problems.

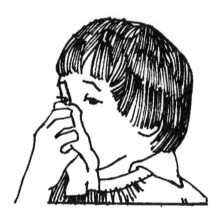

 For older children who can cooperate, have the child blow his or her nose. Hold the unaffected nostril closed.

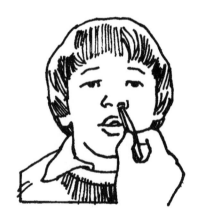

 If the object can be seen near the end of the nostril, and **the child can sit still and upright**, carefully remove the object with tweezers.

  If unsuccessful in removing the object, call your doctor or visit your local hospital emergency department.

PREVENTION

• Keep small objects away from children.

• Supervise children carefully. They frequently put small objects (e.g., food, small toys, stones) into any body opening.

• Teach children not to put small objects into any body opening.

NOTES:

Panic And Anxiety

MAY SEE:
- shortness of breath
- dizziness
- palpitations (heart pounding)
- trembling
- excessive sweating
- stomach pain
- fear of dying

- smothering sensation
- fainting
- increased heart rate
- shaking
- nausea
- chest pain
- feeling out of control

 Do not leave the child alone.

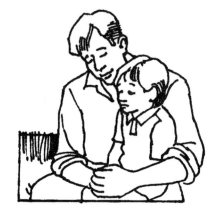

 Stay calm and try to reassure the child.

Assist the child to relax, for example:
- slow, deep breathing
- distraction
- music
- rest

Protect the child from hurting himself or herself.

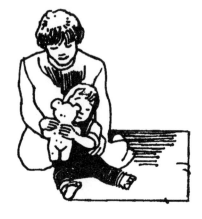

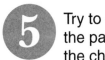 Try to determine the cause of the panic attack. Encourage the child to talk about it.

 Call the doctor if:
- the child is unable to control the attack
- attacks occur repeatedly
- you suspect the cause is physical

PREVENTION:
- Assist the child to learn ways to deal with fears and stress.
- Counselling may help.
- Contact your doctor or a public health nurse for referral.

Poison Ivy *(Poison Oak, Summach)*

MAY SEE: Rash may appear one to three days after contact. It may begin as red swellings and itchiness, and may become weeping blisters occuring in streaks and patches.

 If you know the child has been in contact with poison ivy, flush the affected area immediately with cold, running water.

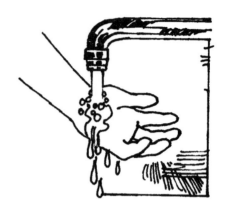

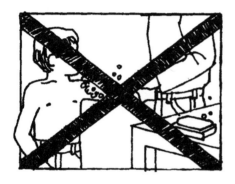

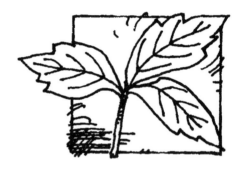

 Do not use soap as it may spread the plant's oils.

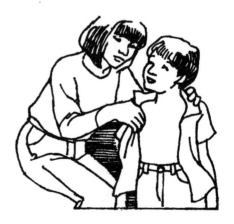

 Remove the child's clothing. Wash the clothing in hot water and detergent.

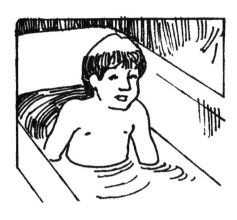

 For itching and discomfort:
- give the child a cool bath
- massage the area with an ice cube
- let the skin air dry
- apply calamine lotion
- keep the child's nails short to discourage scratching

If the skin is blistered, cool salt water compresses (5 mL [1 teaspoon] salt in 500 mL [2 cups] water) are effective.

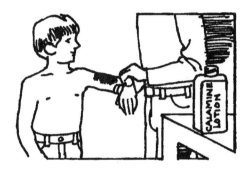

 If the rash is severe, contact your doctor for further treatment.

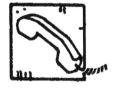

COMMENT:
- Toxins from poisonous plants can remain a hazard for up to a year.

PREVENTION:
- Wear protective clothing when walking in unknown woods and grassy areas.
- Teach children to recognize poisonous plants and stay away from them.
- Change the child's clothing and wash the clothing immediately if exposure is suspected.

Poisons: Eyes

MAY SEE:
- redness
- itching in eyes
- blurred vision or other visual changes
- blindness
- burning
- excessive tearing
- pain in eyes

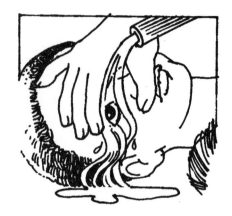

1 Flush the child's eyes with lukewarm water continuously for 15 to 20 minutes.

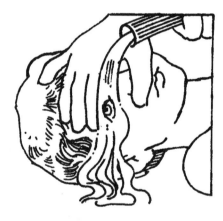

2 Turn the child's head so that the injured eye is down and to the side. Be careful not to flush poison into the other eye.
- hold the child's head under the faucet in a sink or in a shower OR
- pour water into the eye from a pitcher or glass

3 Call the poison control center or visit your local hospital emergency department. An eye exam may be required.

PREVENTION:

- Keep all poisonous substances, aerosol sprays, etc. locked up and away from children.
- Keep the poison control number by the phone, and write the number inside the front cover of this book.
- Teach children the meaning of poison symbols.

NOTES:

Poisons: Inhaled

MAY SEE:
- irritated eyes, nose and throat
- dizziness
- headaches
- bluish color around mouth or nailbeds
- unconsciousness
- coughing
- vomiting
- convulsions
- trouble breathing

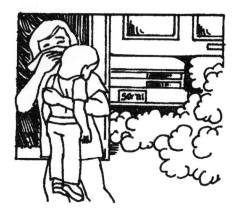

 Remove the child from the poison or fumes.

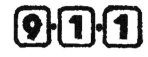

 If the child is having trouble breathing or does not respond, call 9-1-1 or local Emergency Medical Services number. Refer to:

BREATHING/C.P.R.		UNCONSCIOUS	
0 to 1 year	Page 34	0 to 1 year	Page 172
Over 1 year	Page 38	Over 1 year	Page 176

 Protect yourself with a wet cloth over your mouth and nose. Stay below the fumes.

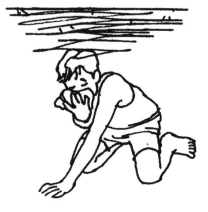

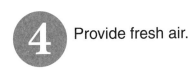
4 Provide fresh air.

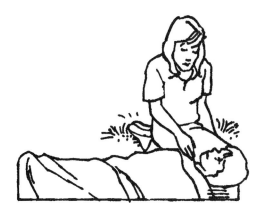

 5 Keep the child warm.

6 Call the poison control center or visit your local hospital emergency department.
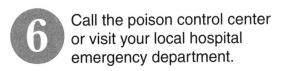

COMMENT:
- Remember, you are also at risk from the fumes. Do not stay in the area for long periods of time when you are attempting to remove the child.

PREVENTION:
- Keep all chemicals locked up away from children.
- Do not leave children alone in running cars.
- Keep the poison control number by the phone, and write the number inside the front cover of this book.
- Install a carbon monoxide sensor in your home.
- Clean and repair chimneys and gas vents at least yearly.
- Have regular gas inspections done by a licensed gas inspector (often employed by utility or plumbing and heating companies).
- Teach children the meanings of chemical warning symbols on containers.

Poisons: Skin

Ensure you are not in contact with poisons while helping the child.

MAY SEE:
- burning and redness of skin
- rash
- swelling
- itchiness
- blisters
- fever

 If the child is having trouble breathing or does not respond, call 9-1-1 or your local Emergency Medical Services number. Refer to:

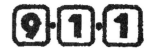

BREATHING/C.P.R.		UNCONSCIOUS	
0 to 1 year	Page 34	0 to 1 year	Page 172
Over 1 year	Page 38	Over 1 year	Page 176

 If burns are severe or on the face, call 9-1-1 or your local Emergency Medical Services number.

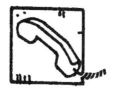

 If the child is not unconscious, identify the poison and call the poison control centre or visit your local hospital emergency department for advice.

 Wearing gloves, remove poisons that are in contact with the skin. Use a clean dry cloth. Throw the cloth away.

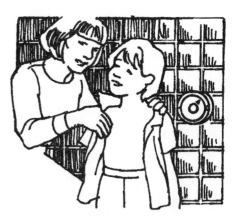

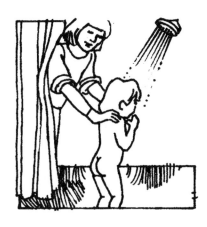

 Flush the child's skin with running water for at least 15 minutes:
- use a shower if needed
- remove the child's clothing and any jewelery while in water
- avoid getting poison in the child's eyes or mouth

 Cover any burned areas with a clean dry cloth or bandage.

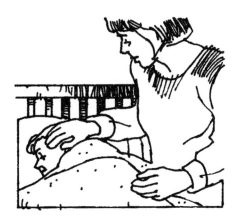

 Keep the child warm.

PREVENTION:
- Keep the poison control number by the phone and write the number inside the front cover of this book.
- Keep all poisons (e.g., chemicals) in a locked cupboard away from children's reach.
- Teach children the meaning of poison symbols.

Poisons: Swallowed

MAY SEE:
- nausea
- diarrhea
- drowsiness
- difficulty breathing
- thirst
- coma
- cramping in stomach
- vomiting
- headaches
- slurred speech
- cool clammy skin
- convulsions
- burning around mouth and lips

 1 If the child is having trouble breathing or does not respond, call 9-1-1 or your local Emergency Medical Service number. Refer to:

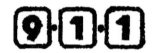

BREATHING/C.P.R.		UNCONSCIOUS	
0 to 1 year	Page 34	0 to 1 year	Page 172
Over 1 year	Page 38	Over 1 year	Page 176

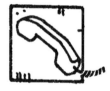

 2 If the child is not unconscious, call the poison control center or visit your local hospital emergency department for advice.

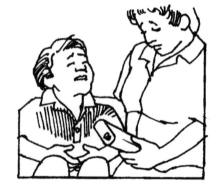

 3 Try to identify the poison. Information on the container label may be helpful.

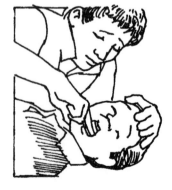

 4 If the child is awake, empty his or her mouth of the substance taken (avoid force to prevent choking).

Only under the advice of the poison centre or a doctor should the child be made to vomit using Syrup of Ipecac, and use only within the first 30 minutes.

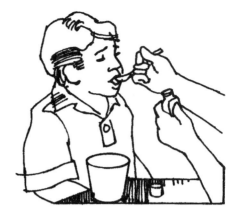

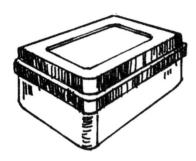

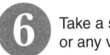 Take a sample of the poison or any vomit to the hospital.

COMMENT:
- Children are curious and they can find poisons in many different areas (e.g., purses, bags, garages, neighbours' houses).

PREVENTION:
- Keep Syrup of Ipecac locked up with other medications.
- Keep the poison control number by the phone and write the number inside the front cover of this book.
- Keep medicine, vitamins and poisons locked up, away from children.
- Do not keep poisonous plants in your home.
- Do not call medicine "candy".
- Keep medicine and vitamins separate from other poisons; all should be locked up away from children.

Scabies

1 Check with your doctor or public health nurse if you are unsure whether or not your child has scabies.

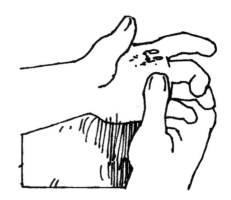

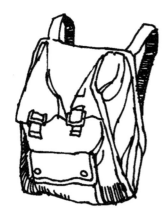

2 Notify the school or day care. They will send home your child's clothes, will clean toys, and make sure others do not have scabies.

3 Buy the lotion suggested by your pharmacist or doctor. Pregnant or nursing women and children under two years old need special treatment.

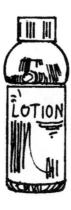

Follow the package instructions carefully.

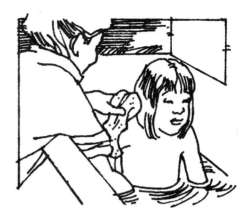

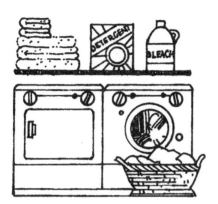

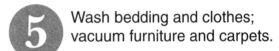

 Wash bedding and clothes; vacuum furniture and carpets.

6 Do not send children to school or day care until 12 hours after the whole family has been treated.

COMMENTS:
- Scabies is a very small bug that burrows under the skin. By the time the rash shows up the bug has been there for four to six weeks.
- This is often mistaken for other skin diseases.
- Children may still feel itchy up to two weeks after treatment. Do not repeat lotion treatment unless advised to do so by your doctor.

Scrapes

MAY SEE:
- Slight scraping of the skin with little bleeding
- possible injury to bone or tissue below

 If serious injury and/or a broken bone is suspected, call your doctor or visit your local hospital emergency department. See **Broken Bones** on page 40.

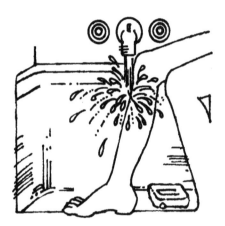

 Clean the area by rinsing with running water; gently remove dirt, etc.

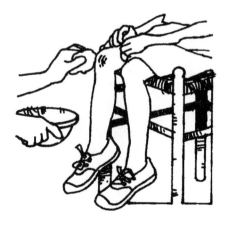 Wash around the area with mild soap and water.

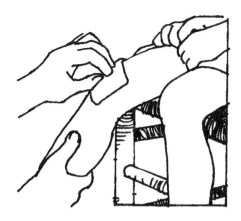

4 Use a clean cloth or towel to dry the scraped area.

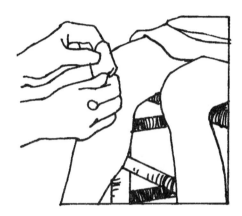

5 Apply a sterile or clean bandage. Keep the scrape clean and dry.

6 Until the scrape is healed, observe for increasing redness, swelling, drainage, pain and/or fever.

COMMENTS:
- Call your doctor or visit your local hospital emergency department as needed.
- To prevent tetanus, be sure that all children are immunized according to your Public or Community Health guidelines.

Shock

MAY SEE:
- cool, clammy, pale skin
- rapid, weak pulse
- weakness
- fast breathing
- anxiety
- pale or blue lips, gums or fingernails

 Call 9-1-1 or your local Emergency Medical Services number.

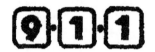

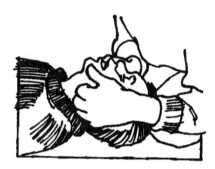

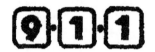 If the child has (or could have) a head or neck injury, see **Head Injuries** page 104. If there is severe external bleeding, attempt to control bleeding; see **Bleeding** on page 74.

 If the child is awake, lay the child in a comfortable position with the legs raised slightly above the level of the chest.

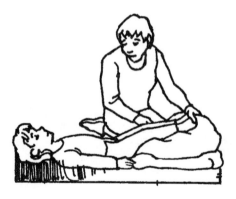

 If the child is experiencing pain in the chest or difficulty breathing, raise the child's head and shoulders.

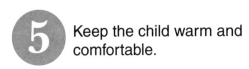 Keep the child warm and comfortable.

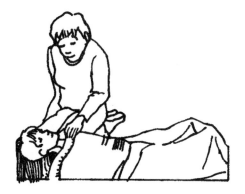

 Do not give the child anything to eat or drink.

COMMENTS:
- Shock is a very serious condition that may be life threatening.
- It can be caused by a number of things such as severe internal or external bleeding, severe dehydration, severe allergic reaction or respiratory failure.

See also:

- **Allergic Reactions** on page 16
- **Dehydration** on page 76
- **Difficulty Breathing** on page 34 (Infants) page 38 (Children)
- **Cuts** on page 74
- **Heat Stroke** on page 112
- **Back and Neck Injuries** on page 20

Sore Throat

MAY SEE:
- complaint of pain in throat
- difficulty breathing
- fever
- difficulty swallowing
- swollen glands in neck

 See your doctor if the child has a sore throat and:

- swollen and/or painful lumps in neck
- drooling, see page 82
- pus (thick yellow or white drainage) from eyes, nose or throat
- chest pain
- stiff neck
- frequent vomiting
- headache
- difficulty in swallowing that worsens quickly, see page 82
- earache
- difficulty breathing
- rash
- extreme weakness and/ or confusion
- abdominal pain

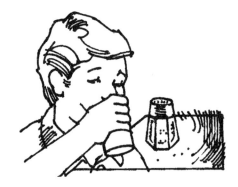

 Give warm, salt-water gargles as needed to provide comfort.

 Give acetaminophen (e.g., Tylenol or Tempra) as per directions on the bottle.

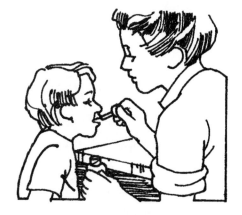

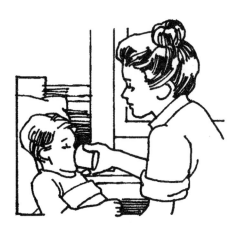

 Encourage rest and extra fluids.

 If sore throat and fever continue beyond 24 to 36 hours, see your doctor.

PREVENTION:
• Do not share dishes, food, drinks or toothbrushes.

• Have everyone in the family wash their hands frequently.

Sprains Or Strains

MAY SEE:
- swelling
- discoloration
- pain
- loss of movement

 Apply ice to the injury immediately. Do not apply ice directly to skin, use a towel or cloth between ice and skin. Apply for 15 to 20 minutes every two hours.

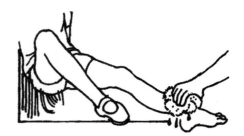

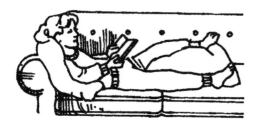 Elevate the injured limb.

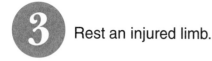 Rest an injured limb.

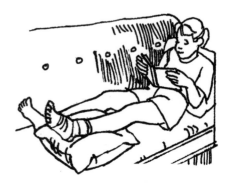

 For discomfort you may use:
- a mild pain reliever (e.g., acetaminophen – Tylenol or Tempra).
- a tensor wrap on the sprained area for support of the limb; do not wrap tightly.

5 Watch the limb for changes in circulation (e.g., tingling, cold, numb, loss of movement, increased pain, pale color or blue color). Contact your doctor if you see any of these signs.

COMMENTS:

• If the child has a great deal of pain, is unable to bear weight, or experiences loss of movement, see your doctor or visit your local hospital emergency department.

• If the symptoms persist, call or see your doctor for further advice.

Stings *(Bee Or Wasp)*

MAY SEE:

Mild Reaction
(lasts less than 24 to 48 hours)
- redness
- pain
- swelling of two to five centimeters
  (one to two inches)
  around the bite area

Severe Reaction
- rash
- itchiness
- swelling of eyelids, lips,
  tongue and/or throat
- hives
- wheezing
- difficulty breathing

 If the child has difficulty breathing or sudden and severe onset of swelling or hives, call 9-1-1 or your local Emergency Medical Services number. Refer to:

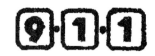

BREATHING/C.P.R.		UNCONSCIOUS	
0 to 1 year	Page 34	0 to 1 year	Page 172
Over 1 year	Page 38	Over 1 year	Page 176

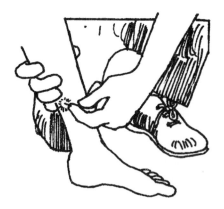

 Remove the stinger, if present, by gently scraping the stinger with a fingernail. Do not squeeze.

 Cleanse the area with soap and water.

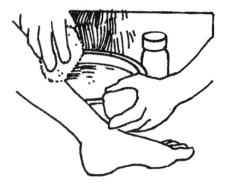

Call your doctor if problems arise (e.g., infection at site). Look for fever, redness, red streaks, discharge, warmth and swelling.

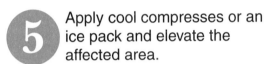 Apply cool compresses or an ice pack and elevate the affected area.

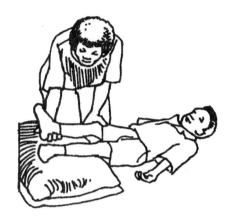

PREVENTION:

• All children should wear shoes outdoors.

• Children who have had a severe reaction should carry a bee sting kit (containing epinephrine). Caregivers should be familiar with emergency treatment.

• Additional measures should be taken to avoid stings (e.g., avoid bright, flowery clothing, perfumes, hairsprays and colognes).

Stomach Ache

MAY SEE: • Pain in the stomach area accompanied by nausea and vomiting, fever, diarrhea or constipation and problems urinating.

• If you suspect **Constipation,** see page 68.

 Contact your doctor or local hospital emergency department if:
• pain is severe, with or without vomiting, lasting more than 1/2 hour
• pain is accompanied by fever or severe diarrhea
• pain occurs repeatedly or pain increases

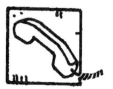

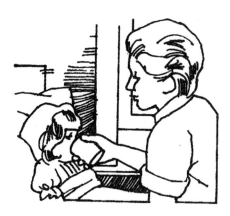

 Comfort the child. Allow only clear fluids, but no milk or food, until the stomach ache passes.

 Do not apply cold or heat to the stomach.

 Do not give the child a laxative or an enema without the advice of a physician.

COMMENTS:

Sometimes stomach ache is a sign of APPENDICITIS which requires immediate medical attention. Symptoms may be:

- mild fever
- loss of appetite
- pain around the belly button and/or right lower stomach (abdomen)
- vomiting
- change in bowel movements
- continuous crying in an infant

- Stomach ache may also be caused by tiredness, overeating, indigestion, food allergies, or minor emotional stress. More serious causes include food poisoning, strep throat, physical injury or pneumonia.

NOTES:

Suicidal Behavior

MAY SEE: Patterns of behavior which may include:

- withdrawal from family and friends
- isolation from others
- agitation/loss of rational thought
- wide mood swings
- sudden cheerfulness following a depression
- poor school performance
- looks sad with little expression
- change in appearance and cleanliness
- eating problems (stops eating or eats excessively)
- talking about harming oneself
- sleep problems (trouble sleeping or always tired, excessive sleeping)
- loss of energy and interest in things
- recurrent headaches and stomach aches
- acting out behavior (unexplained alcohol or drug use, fighting, running away)
- talking about worthlessness and hopelessness
- preoccupied with death
- giving away possessions
- making a will
- lack of concentration
- talking about suicide
- hoarding pills and weapons

**TAKE ALL SUICIDE THREATS SERIOUSLY.
DO NOT BELIEVE IT IS "JUST TO GET ATTENTION".**

 Ask direct questions about depression or suicide threats (e.g., "Are you thinking about suicide?").

 Use a calm approach. Let the child know you care and want to help. Don't give quick advice (e.g., "Everything will be okay.").

 Stay with the child, do not leave him or her alone. If the child runs, call the police immediately.

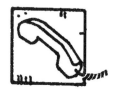

Keep the child safe. Remove pills, guns, ropes, sharp objects, keys.

  Contact professional help or go to your local hospital emergency department. Do not try to handle this on your own. Call the police, crisis line, "Kid's Help Phone" in Canada, public health nurse, or your family physician.

COMMENTS:

Risk factors may include:

- depression
- recent conflict or loss
- break-up with a girlfriend or boyfriend
- death of a friend or family member
- suicide of a friend or family member

- alcohol and drug abuse
- divorce
- family fight or separation
- unplanned pregnancy
- separation/divorce of parents

PREVENTION:

- Control access to prescribed and over-the-counter medications to all children.
- Encourage children to talk openly about their feelings.
- Take an active interest in your children's activities, friends and school.
- Help your child to develop a positive self-esteem.
- KID'S HELP PHONE: 1-800-668-6868 in Canada.

Sunburn

MAY SEE:
- tender, red, swollen skin
- swelling
- burning sensation
- pain
- blisters

 Remove the child from the sun immediately.

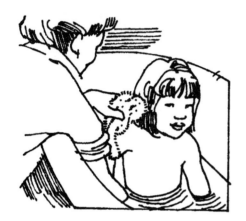

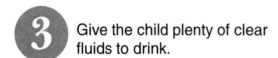 Apply tepid, wet cloths or place the child in a tepid bath until the pain is relieved.

Give the child plenty of clear fluids to drink.

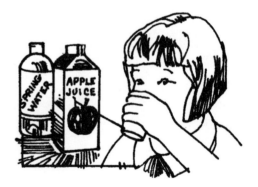

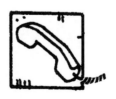 DO NOT BREAK BLISTERS. Contact your doctor for advice.

5 DO NOT APPLY OINTMENT
unless prescribed by a doctor.

  If sunburn is accompanied by symptoms of illness like weakness, chills, fever, paleness, dizziness, nausea, call your doctor or visit your local hospital emergency department. For further information, see **Heat Exhaustion** on page 110, or **Heat Stroke** on page112.

PREVENTIONS

- Use a sunscreen with an SPF of 15 or higher on children over six months of age.

- Apply sunscreen one half hour prior to sun exposure. Reapply every three to four hours.

- Children should wear hats, sunglasses, loose-fitting shirts and pants.

- Children should drink plenty of fluids.

- Children should avoid prolonged exposure to the sun between 10:00 a.m. and 3:00 p.m.

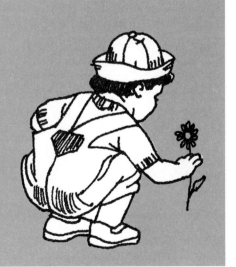

Swallowed Objects

MAY SEE:
- no obvious signs of distress
- pain
- anxiety
- drooling
- difficulty swallowing
- difficulty breathing

 Make sure the child is able to breathe. If the child is having difficulty breathing, call 9-1-1 or your local Emergency Medical Services number. See:

BREATHING/C.P.R.		CHOKING & BREATHING	
0 to 1 year	Page 34	0 to 1 year	Page 58
Over 1 year	Page 38	Over 1 year	Page 60

 If there is difficulty swallowing, go to your local hospital emergency department immediately.

 Some foreign objects, like coins, cause no harm and pass through the intestinal tract in the child's bowel movement.

 No matter what is swallowed, you should seek medical attention for proper follow up.

COMMENTS:

- Remember your ABC's (A = Airway, B = Breathing, C = Circulation/Pulse).
- CPR is a very difficult skill to master. You should enroll in a CPR class. For more information call your local community college, The Red Cross, St. John Ambulance or the Heart and Stroke Foundation.

PREVENTION:
An ounce of prevention is worth a pound of cure

- Cut food into small pieces and make sure infants or children chew food well.
- Popcorn, nuts, small candies should not be given to infants or children.
- Foods such as grapes, spaghetti, wieners, etc. should be cut into small chewable pieces.
- Infants or children should sit down to eat, never allow them to run around while eating.
- Always place infants or children in a car seat in the rear seat while riding in vehicles.
- Make sure all toys have secure pieces (e.g., eyes of stuffed animals won't pull off).
- Infants or children should wear helmets while in bicycle carriers or trailers.
- Cover electrical outlets.
- Keep children away from workshop areas.
- Keep matches out of infants' or children's reach.
- Make sure all medications and/or poisons are in a safe locked place.
- Keep balloons and rubber gloves away from infants or children.
- Keep drapery strings and any cords out of infants' or children's reach.
- Do not dress infants or children in clothing with a drawstring, hood or scarf when they may be playing on play structures.
- Make sure toilet seats are down.
- Keep small, shiny objects out of infants' or children's reach (e.g., coins, earrings, marbles).

Swallowed Objects

Teething

MAY SEE:
- crying
- red or white areas on gums
- red cheeks
- swollen gums
- fever

 Offer a clean, firm, cold object such as a teething ring for the child to bite on. This may help the tooth cut through the gum.

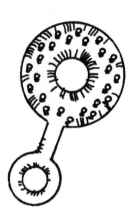

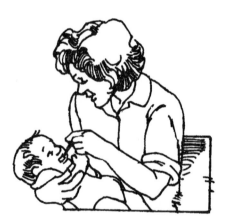

 Acetaminophen (e.g., Tylenol or Tempra) may be used for short-term pain relief. (Aspirin is not recommended, see Aspirin note on page 99.)

If the child develops a fever, see **Fever** page 98.

PREVENTION:
- Do not use foods such as carrots or pickles for teething as they may break off and cause choking.
- Always watch a teething child closely while the child has any type of teething biscuits.

NOTES:

Ticks

 Cover the tick with gauze soaked in mineral oil or petroleum jelly (Vaseline) to cut off the air supply to the tick.

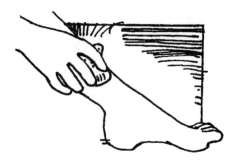

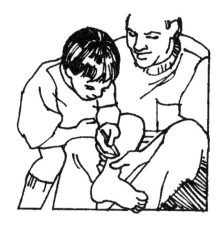

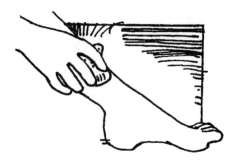 Within half an hour, the tick should let go. Use tweezers and pull up with steady, even pressure to remove the tick and all of its parts.

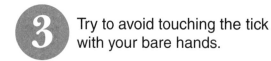 Try to avoid touching the tick with your bare hands.

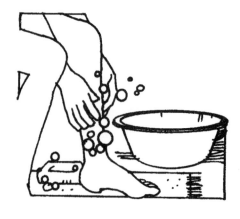

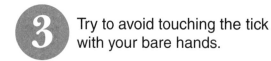 Wash the bite area and your hands with soap and water following tick removal.

COMMENTS:

- If the child develops a fever or rash within ten days after a tick bite, seek immediate medical attention. There is a possiblity of developing Lyme Disease. If you are not sure you have removed all of the tick, contact your doctor.

PREVENTION:

- Children should be checked frequently after outdoor activities where ticks are present.

- Avoid long grass, bushes and woods.

- Wear long sleeves, pants and hats if in the above areas.

- Keep the child's hair tucked under his or her hat.

- Apply insect repellents, containing Deet, but not on babies or children under one year.

NOTES:

Toothaches

 Rinse the child's mouth vigorously with warm water to clean out debris.

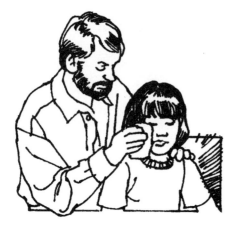

2 Apply cold compresses to the child's face over the aching tooth.

3 You may give the child acetaminophen (e.g., Tylenol or Tempra) for pain relief.

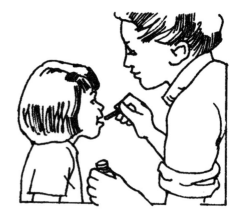

4 Do not put acetaminophen directly on the tooth or gum tissue.

5 Consult your dentist for an examination and advice.

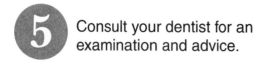

COMMENT:

• If the child develops a high fever, consult your doctor.

PREVENTION:

• Visit your dentist regularly.

• Brush young children's teeth at bedtime and following meals; older children should be encouraged to brush regularly.

• Floss young children's teeth daily; older children should be encouraged to floss regularly.

• Do not let your child fall asleep with a bottle of juice or milk in his or her mouth.

• Wipe a baby's mouth out with a wet cloth following feeding.

• Limit sugar-rich foods.

• Use fluoride as recommended by your doctor or dentist.

NOTES:

Tooth Injuries

1 Gently clean any dirt or debris from the injured area with warm water.

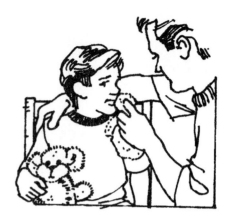

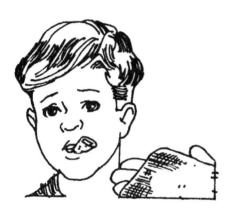

2 Apply cold compresses or an ice pack to the child's face over the injured tooth to keep the swelling down.

3 If the injured tooth is permanent, and it appears to be a clean break, rinse the tooth gently in running water, but do not scrub.

4 Place the tooth back in the socket.

5 If it is not possible to place the tooth back in the socket, place it in a container of milk.

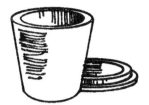

6 Take the child to your dentist immediately.

COMMENT:
- If the child is taken to the dentist within 30 minutes of injury, the chances of successful replanting are fair. For all tooth injuries, take the child to the dentist immediately.

PREVENTION:
- Use a mouth guard for contact sports.

Trapped: Confined Spaces

These include: • silos   • cisterns/wells
                 • refrigerators/freezers

 Confined spaces such as silos, cisterns and wells do not contain enough oxygen to sustain life. NEVER ENTER THESE SPACES WITHOUT APPROPRIATE RESCUE GEAR AND SELF-CONTAINED BREATHING APPARATUS.

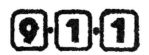 Call 9-1-1 or your local Emergency Medical Services number.

 Once the child is safely rescued, check for breathing. If the child is not breathing turn to:

BREATHING/C.P.R.		UNCONSCIOUS	
0 to 1 year	Page 34	0 to 1 year	Page 172
Over 1 year	Page 38	Over 1 year	Page 176

PREVENTION:

- Ensure all safety devices are working and in place.
- Never leave a child unsupervised.
- Educate your child about local hazards and safety procedures.
- Remove doors from unused refrigerators or freezers.

NOTES:

Unconscious: Infants *(Newborn To 1 Year)*

MAY SEE:
- pale or bluish colour
- unresponsive (will not wake up)
- not breathing
- limpness

 Establish unresponsiveness by gently tapping the infant's feet and hands. DO NOT SHAKE.

 DO NOT LEAVE THE INFANT. If not responsive (not waking up) and you are not alone, have someone call 9-1-1 or your local Emergency Medical Services number.

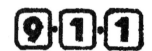

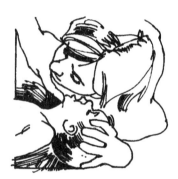

AIRWAY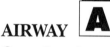
Open the airway by gently tilting the head back with one hand and lifting the chin with the other hand.

If you suspect a neck injury due to a fall or a motor vehicle accident, etc., carefully perform the chin lift to avoid twisting the neck.

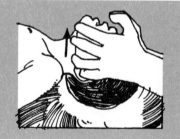

4 CHECK FOR BREATHING FOR THREE TO FIVE SECONDS
- **Look** to see if chest/stomach is moving
- **Listen** for sounds of breathing
- **Feel** for air on your cheek.

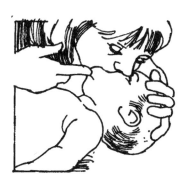

5 **BREATHING**
Give two breaths of air by covering the mouth and nose with your mouth. If air does not enter with the first breath, reposition the head and try to breathe for the infant again.

DOES THE STOMACH AND CHEST RISE WITH BREATH?

NO: **(If YES, turn to the next page.)**

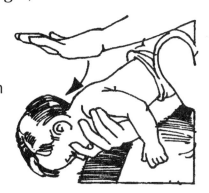

6 If the airway is blocked, give up to five back blows, between the shoulder blades, using the heel of your hand, followed by up to five chest thrusts.

Chest Thrust Landmarks:
- Draw an imaginary line between the two nipples.
- Move three fingers towards the middle of the chest with your index (pointer) finger touching that line.
- Lift the index (pointer) finger and press down one-half to one inch with two fingers (you should be on the lower part of the breast bone – one finger width below the imaginary line).

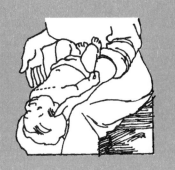

Check the airway. **Only** if you **see** the object, use your fingers to "sweep" the object. If the object is not visible, continue back blows and chest thrusts.

Continued Next Page

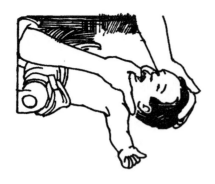

 AIRWAY

Grab the chin and tongue with one hand and pull forward (Tongue/Jaw Lift). Look in the mouth. ONLY if you see an object in the mouth, gently sweep the mouth with two fingers to remove the object.

 Repeat steps five to seven until effective or ambulance arrives.

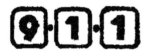

- IF AIRWAY REMAINS BLOCKED AND YOU ARE STILL ALONE, take the infant with you and call 9-1-1 or your local Emergency Medical Services number after one minute of rescue breathing.
- If blockage is removed, check pulse.
- IF INFANT STARTS BREATHING place him or her on one side.
- If no pulse, perform C.P.R.:

BREATHING/C.P.R.	
0 to 1 year	Page 34
Over 1 year	Page 38

DOES THE STOMACH AND CHEST RISE WITH BREATHING?

YES:

 IF YOU ARE ABLE TO GET AIR INTO THE AIRWAY, BUT THE INFANT IS STILL UNCONSCIOUS (SLEEPING) perform rescue breaths at a rate of one breath every three seconds or 20 breaths per minute.

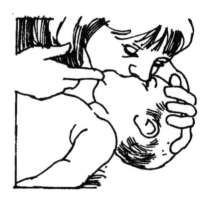

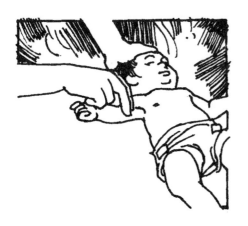

7 **CIRCULATION**

Check for pulse – if none perform C.P.R. See:

BREATHING/C.P.R.	
0 to 1 year	Page 34
Over 1 year	Page 38

COMMENTS:

An ounce of prevention is worth a pound of cure.

- Keep small objects away from infants.
- Keep small, shiny objects out of infants' reach (e.g., coins, earrings, marbles).
- Cut food into small pieces and make sure infants chew food well.
- Foods such as grapes, spaghetti, wieners, etc. should always be cut into small, chewable pieces.
- Popcorn, nuts, small candies should not be given to small infants.
- Infants should sit down to eat, never allow them to run around while eating.
- Make sure all toys have secure pieces (e.g., eyes of stuffed animals won't pull off).
- Keep infants away from workshop areas.
- Keep balloons and rubber gloves away from infants.
- Keep drapery strings and any cords out of infants' reach.

Unconscious: Children (Over 1 Year)

MAY SEE:
- unresponsive
- not breathing
- pale or bluish in colour
- limpness

 DO NOT LEAVE THE CHILD. If you are not alone, have someone call 9-1-1 or your local Emergency Medical Services number.

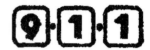

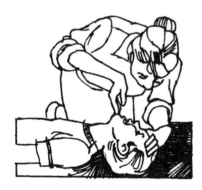

 AIRWAY **A**
Open airway by gently tilting the head back with one hand and lifting the chin with the other hand.

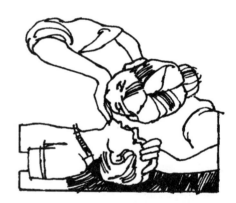

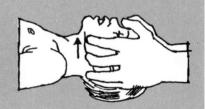 CHECK FOR BREATHING FOR THREE TO FIVE SECONDS
- **Look** to see if the chest/stomach is moving
- **Listen** for sounds of breathing
- **Feel** for air on your cheek

If you suspect a neck injury due to a fall or a motor vehicle accident, etc., carefully perform the chin lift to avoid twisting the neck.

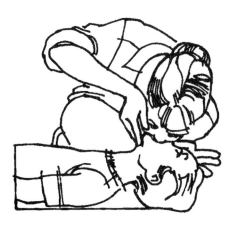

BREATHING **B**

4 Give two breaths of air. If child is small, you may need to cover the nose and mouth with your mouth. If air does not enter with the first breath, reposition the head and try to breathe for the child again.

DOES THE STOMACH AND CHEST RISE WITH BREATH?

NO: (If YES, turn to the next page.)

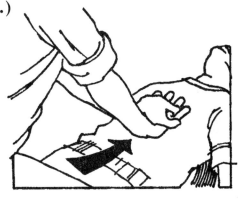

5 If the airway is blocked, give up to five abdominal thrusts by placing the heel of one hand just above the belly button and thrust inward and upward.

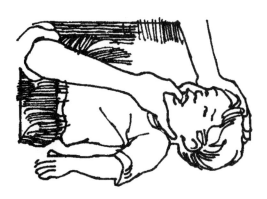

AIRWAY **A**

6 Grab the chin and tongue with one hand and pull forward (Tongue/Jaw Lift). Look in the mouth. ONLY if you see an object in the mouth, gently sweep the mouth with two fingers to remove the object.

7 Repeat steps four to six until effective or ambulance arrives.

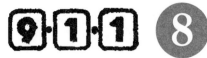 **8** IF THE AIRWAY REMAINS BLOCKED AND YOU ARE STILL ALONE, take the child with you and call 9-1-1 or your local Emergency Medical Services number.

DOES THE STOMACH AND CHEST RISE WITH BREATHING?

YES:

5 Breath for the child, one breath every three seconds or 20 breaths per minute.

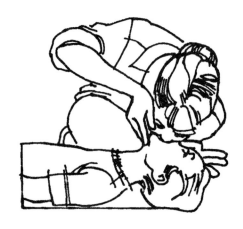

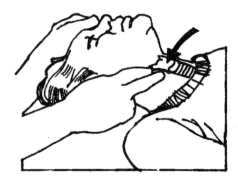

6 CIRCULATION

Check pulse. If no pulse, start CPR. See:

BREATHING/C.P.R.	
0 to 1 year	Page 34
Over 1 year	Page 38

7
- IF YOU ARE ABLE TO GET AIR INTO THE AIRWAY, BUT THE CHILD IS STILL UNCONSCIOUS (SLEEPING) perform rescue breaths at a rate of one breath every three seconds or 20 breaths per minute.

- IF THE CHILD STARTS BREATHING place him or her on one side.

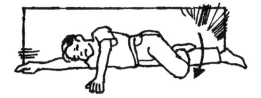

COMMENTS:

An ounce of prevention is worth a pound of cure.

- Keep small objects away from children.

- Keep small, shiny objects out of children's reach (e.g., coins, earrings, marbles).

- Popcorn, nuts, small candies should not be given to small children.

- Goods such as grapes, spaghetti, wieners, etc. should be cut into small, chewable pieces.

- Children should sit down to eat, never allow them to run around while eating.

- Make sure all toys have secure pieces (e.g., eyes of stuffed animals won't pull off).

- Keep children away from workshop areas.

- Keep balloons and rubber gloves away from small children.

- Keep drapery strings and any cords out of children's reach.

Urination Pain

MAY SEE:

In Infants and Toddlers
- colic
- bad-smelling urine
- poor feeding
- fever
- vomiting

In Children Over Two Years
- fever
- bad-smelling urine
- stomach ache
- frequent urination
- urination pain

 Have the child examined by a doctor as soon as possible.

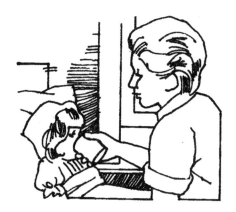

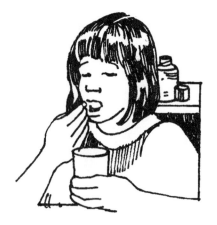 Encourage the child to drink lots of fluids.

A mild pain reliever like acetaminophen (e.g., Tylenol or Tempra) given as directed may help with the pain.

COMMENT:
• Painful urination is most commonly caused by injury or infection.

PREVENTION:
• Good hygiene is important.

• Teach young girls to clean from front to back following urination.

• Encourage children to empty their bladders fully.

• Older boys should be taught to cleanse underneath foreskin if it retracts easily.

NOTES:

Vomiting

 Offer the child small amounts of clear fluids frequently. Use oral rehydration products like: Pedialyte or Gastrolyte for small children; flat ginger ale and popsicles for older children. Give the child one ounce every hour for three to four hours and gradually increase if the child tolerates well.

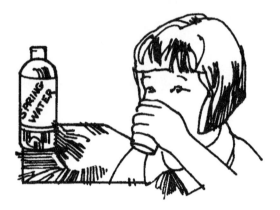 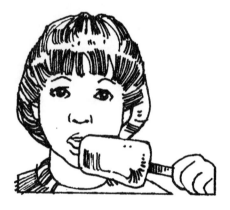

 Do not give the child milk, food or large amounts of fluid until vomiting stops.

 Observe for signs of dehydration:
- child's eyes dark and sunken
- child becomes listless, drowsy or confused
- decreased urination/wet diapers
- dry lips
- sunken soft spot on a baby's head
- crying without tear
- refusing fluids

See **Dehydration** page 76

COMMENTS:

Always contact your doctor if:
- the child continues to vomit frequently
- the child shows any signs of dehydration
- vomiting is accompanied by frequent diarrhea in a small child
- vomit contains blood or looks like coffee grounds
- vomiting is accompanied by high fever, severe headache or severe abdominal pain lasting more than 30 minutes
- an infant vomits, especially if it is repeated and/or forceful
- vomiting occurs after a head injury or a convulsion
- the child's stomach is hard and bloated in between episodes of vomiting

NOTES:

Weight Loss: Anorexia Nervosa

MAY SEE:

Patterns of behavior which may include:

- little or no food intake
- focus on food (talking about food, preparing food for others, shopping for food)
- frequent compulsive exercise
- withdrawal from others
- child feels fat even when thin
- baggy clothes to cover weight loss
- vomiting after eating (e.g., going into the bathroom after a meal)
- loss of menstruation
- irritability
- depression

With extreme weight loss, you may see:

- dizziness
- paleness
- dry skin and hair
- slow or irregular heart beat
- fainting
- cold (especially hands and feet)
- brittle nails
- convulsions

 Do not argue with the child about food, weight or appearance, it will only push the child away.

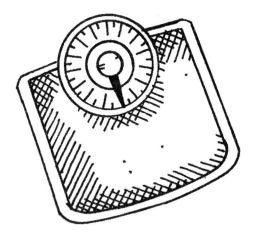

 Use a calm, caring and firm approach to take the child to help.

3 Get professional help. Call any of the following: your family doctor, nutritionist, public health nurse, local eating disorder clinic, counsellor, child psychiatrist.

COMMENT:
- If symptoms are accompanied by signs of severe illness, call your doctor immediately or visit your local hospital emergency department.

NOTES:

NOTES:

CHILDREN'S WELLNESS

SECTION

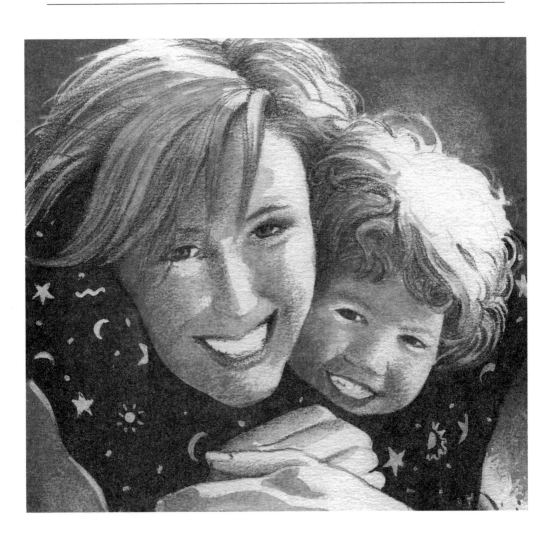

Feeding: Infants *(Newborn To 1 Year)*

Breast feeding is the best way to feed a new baby. It helps protect your baby from infections and allergies, and gives your baby the best nutrition possible. The only vitamin a breast-fed baby needs is vitamin D.

Breast feeding may be difficult at first, but it gets easier as the first month passes. Ask for support and help from:

- family
- public health nurse
- La Leche League
- friends
- lactation consultant
- family doctor

 Until your baby is four months old, the only food needed is breast milk and vitamin D, or formula. If you are thinking of starting other foods or liquids, talk to your public health nurse or doctor first.

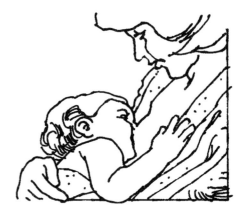

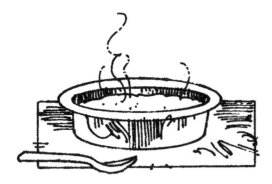

Between four and six months, you will want to start iron-fortified infant cereals. Start with a single grain like rice, before trying mixed cereals. Serve food lukewarm. Your baby may spit out the cereal at first.

 Around six or seven months, you can start vegetables, then fruits. Try one new food every four to five days before trying the next one, in case of allergies. Do not force a food if your infant does not seem to like it, try it again in a few weeks.

4 Babies should get their nutrition from breast milk or formula and baby foods. **Limit your baby to two ounces of half-strength juice each day**, to avoid unnecessary sugar.

5 *By about eight or nine months* your child can start eating foods with a thicker, more lumpy texture. Try meats and poultry.

6 *At one year old* you can introduce egg whites. Your child will now likely eat table foods. You can switch to homogenized milk at this time, but it is much too early for 2% milk. Young children need some fat in their diets for proper brain development.

NOTES:

Feeding: Children (Over 1 Year)

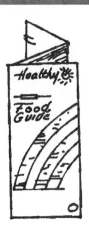

1 Offer your children a variety of foods from all four food groups.

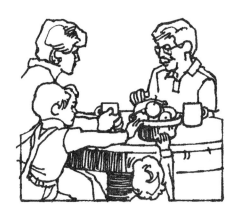

2 Allow your child to decide the number of servings they want to eat, keeping within the number recommended in the Canada or U.S. Food Guide.

3 To avoid choking, do not serve chewing gum, popcorn, raisins, nuts, whole grapes or round wiener slices to children under four years of age.

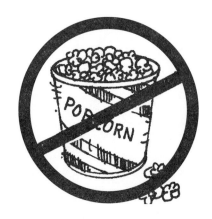

MAKING MEAL TIME PLEASANT:

- Schedule meals and snacks at regular times.

- Children as young as two years old can participate in simple food preparation like scrubbing a potato. This increases their willingness to try different foods.

- Do not insist that children eat if they are not hungry.

- Give children small portions with the option for seconds.

DON'T WORRY IF YOUR CHILD:

- Liked a certain food yesterday, but not today.

- Eats poorly for several days, but then makes up for it on others.

- Refuses food for reasons that seem silly (e.g., the gravy touched the peas).

REMEMBER!

- Offer healthy foods, but give your child the choice to refuse, or to select portion size. As long as they only have access to healthy foods, they will get the nutrition they need.

- Don't get into power struggles.

- Don't bribe children to eat.

For help or more information, call your Public or Community Health department, nurse, nutritionist or doctor.

Immunization And Your Child

WHAT IS IMMUNIZATION?
- Immunization involves giving vaccine that helps protect people against certain diseases.
- Before there was immunization, many children became very sick and some died from these diseases.

WHO SHOULD BE IMMUNIZED?
- All children should be fully immunized at all times.
- While these diseases are less common today, there are still risks. Children can still get these diseases.
- If an epidemic occurs, children not immunized against that disease may be asked to stay out of school or daycare.
- In some provinces or states and countries, children must be immunized before they can go to school or daycare.

WHAT DISEASES WILL MY CHILD BE IMMUNIZED AGAINST?
- In the first years of life, your child will be immunized and protected against the following diseases:
  - diphtheria
  - tetanus
  - lock jaw
  - pertussis (whooping cough)
  - polio
  - haemophilus disease
  - measles
  - mumps
  - rubella (German measles)
- In many areas, your child will be able to receive Hepatitis B vaccine at school.
- New vaccines may also become available for other diseases.

WHEN SHOULD MY CHILD BE IMMUNIZED?
- You should take your child to be immunized at the following ages:
  - two, four, six, 12 and 18 months of age
  - four years of age
  - 10 or 11 years of age
  - 13 or 14 years of age
- Children are better protected when immunized at the recommended times.
- Children also benefit from immunization even if it's late.

WHEN SHOULD MY CHILD NOT BE IMMUNIZED?

- If your child has a fever (more than 38.5°C [101.3°F]), he or she should not be immunized.
- Your child can be immunized if he or she has an ordinary cold or runny nose.
- Allergies are rarely a problem for immunization. You should discuss this with your public health nurse or doctor.
- Your nurse or doctor will let you know if your child should not be immunized.

QUICK FACTS:

- Immunization protects people from many serious diseases.
- Children benefit from immunization even if it's late.
- Keep permanent records of all immunizations.

NOTES:

Parenting: What Is Discipline?

- Discipline is a part of parenting that helps your children learn how to get along with others, learn appropriate behavior and avoid problems as they get older.

- Parents who use discipline well also help their children to feel good about themselves and to learn how to take care of themselves.

- Discipline is not meant to be punishment; it is loving children enough to try to correct their behavior.

- Children often misbehave when they are tired, hungry, sick, angry, jealous, afraid or upset. Understanding this can help you decide how to help them change their behavior.

TO ENCOURAGE GOOD BEHAVIOR:

- Give your child hugs, kisses and praise for good behavior.

- Respect your child by really listening to him or her and asking questions.

- Try to understand your children's point of view, and why they behave as they do.

- Let children make choices that are safe for their ages. Try to increase their choices and responsibilities as they get older.

- Be a good example.

TO AVOID MISBEHAVIOR:

- Only have rules about things that are important but be consistent about those rules. Be fair but firm.

- Don't make empty threats that you can't or don't intend to keep. Children know that they can ignore these threats and you too!

- Make sure children know the reason for a rule, and what will happen if it's broken. Follow through on the consequence.

- Control your emotions. Wait until you're calm to deal with a problem.

- Never insult or humiliate your children.

ALTERNATIVES TO HITTING:

• Remove privileges, toys or entertainment, but not love. Be reasonable with this so you are able to follow through (e.g., don't say "I'll never bring you here again." if you know that you will).

• Remove your child from a situation which is a problem. The child might go to his or her room or sit in a corner to cool off. Make sure the child is safe, and knows how long to stay there. The time should be reasonable for the age (e.g., five years old, five minutes; ten years old, ten minutes). Talk with your child after the child is allowed out.

• Have your child repair or replace a broken item. The child should "work" to pay for it and apologize to the owner.

AVOID HITTING CHILDREN:

• This can easily become a habit that sets a bad example to your children.

• It can lead to child abuse.

• It often takes the place of better, more effective approaches.

• Try just placing your hand firmly on your child's shoulder while you choose a better way to discipline.

HELP IS EASILY FOUND:

• Don't be afraid to ask for suggestions or hints from community agencies or your public health nurse.

What Every Child Needs

- Children don't come with parent training manuals.
- Make the effort to **learn** to be a good parent.
- Classes are offered at community centers, libraries, health departments and many other agencies.

LOVE:

- is to know that someone cares about him or her very much

  Try saying - "I love you."
  - "I really enjoyed doing that with you."
  - "I love your sense of humor."

ACCEPTANCE:

- is to know that they are "good enough" just the way they are

  Try saying - "You did a good job on that."
  - "Thanks, I really appreciated that."
  - "I'm sure you'll do well."

SECURITY:

- is to know that home is a good, safe place; that someone will always "be there" for him or her

GUIDANCE:

- is to learn how to behave, and that there are limits which must be respected

  Try - setting an example of how you want him or her to act
  - setting reasonable rules and holding him or her to them

Children At Home On Their Own

- children under 12 should NEVER be left alone
- be aware of the laws specific to your area

Here are some tips for teenagers, to make being home alone a positive experience.

PARENTS:
Household Rules:
- stay in the house or yard
- don't invite or have other people in the house when parents are not home
- don't talk to strangers

Emergencies:
- prepare your children to handle all kinds of emergencies/problems
- review fire procedures and local emergency telephone numbers e.g., (9-1-1)

First Aid:
- with your child(ren), assemble a first aid kit
- teach children how to handle burns, bites and bleeding

Phone Lists:
- a phone list, like the one on the inside cover of this book, should be beside each phone in the house
- children should have a neighbour to contact in case of emergencies

CHILDREN:
House Key:
- always carry your key on you
- the best place for your key is around your neck on a chain or string
- keep it out of sight

Strangers:
- strangers are people you don't know, even if you see them every day
- don't talk to strangers and never let them know you are at home alone
- don't answer the door unless you know the person at the door

House Rules:
- follow the house rules that you and your parents have agreed on

Emergencies/Problems:
- make sure you know what to do in each likely emergency situation

Phone:
- don't let a caller know your parents are not home

Fitness

Studies have shown:

- children spend 25 to 30 hours each week sitting in school.
- the average child watches more than 16 hours of television each week.
- children today are up to 40 percent less active than children were 30 years ago.
- daily exercise helps children physically, helps them in school and helps them deal with stress.

 You can help your child have an active lifestyle by:
- enrolling him or her in activities and sports
- building activity into your family lifestyle (e.g., take a walk every night after supper)
- monitor the amount of television watched, and limit if necessary

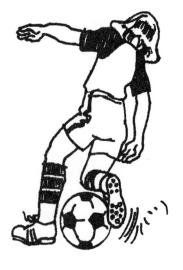

 Daily exercise could include:
- biking
- swimming
- dancing
- skipping
- walking, hiking, running
- team sports
- active, outdoor games
- skating

Television Viewing

A number of studies have shown that children watch approximately 26 hours of television per week.

Some researchers have also studied the effects of television violence on aggressive behaviour in children.

Here are some tips on how to use the television to your advantage:

1. Place time limits on the amount of television your children watch

2. Never use television or videos as a baby sitter.

3. Watch television with your children so you can explain to them:
    • the parts they don't understand
    • what is real and what is not
    • what is right and what is wrong

4. Be aware that children's programs, even cartoons, often have more violence in them than adult programs.

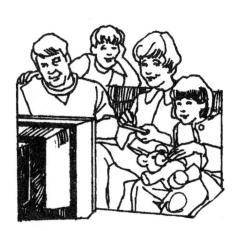

5. Television viewing robs children of their play time. It is through play that children often learn social skills and develop creativity.

6. Educational programs like *Sesame Street* or *Mr. Rogers' Neighborhood* can actually teach your child and help your child's development.

Household Safety

Our homes should be safe places for children, but they are often the place where accidents and injuries are most likely to happen. The most common types of injuries include:

- burns
- falls
- electric shocks
- poisoning
- choking/suffocation

Most of these accidents could be prevented by planning ahead and making your home safe.

BURNS:

- install smoke detectors and replace batteries twice a year
- have a fire extinguisher and check it annually
- keep cigarettes and matches away from children
- keep children away from the stove, have pot handles turned in
- do not drink hot liquids while holding babies or children
- teach children a fire safety plan and practice yearly
- keep your water heater set on "low" or 49° C (120° F)
- always check bath water before placing children in tub
- always turn hot water on last and off first

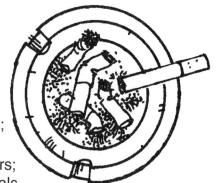

POISONING:

- keep all vitamins and medication in a locked cupboard, out of climbing reach
- do not call vitamins or medicine "candy"
- go through each room of the house to identify and safely store chemicals and poisons
- install carbon monoxide detectors in your home
- dispose of "empty" containers in a garbage can that kids can't get into
- keep house plants out of reach of small children; many house plants are poisonous
- always store chemicals in their original containers; never use food containers to store other chemicals
- keep all ashtrays, cigarettes and alcoholic drinks out of reach of children; alcohol and nicotine can poison kids
- teach children to understand and respect the poison warning symbols on containers

FALLS:

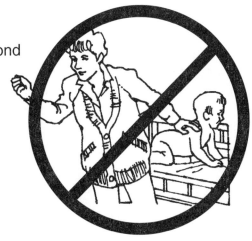

- never turn your back on a baby on a bed, couch or change table, not even for a second
- make sure crib rails are securely up before leaving
- always use the belts on high chairs, strollers and grocery carts
- use properly installed child gates at the top and bottom of all stairs
- all windows and balcony doors need child-proof latches
- never leave a child alone on a balcony

CHOKING/SUFFOCATION:

- Keep dangerous items out of reach of children under four years of age; this includes:

  - plastic bags and plastic wrap
  - broken crayons and toys
  - safety pins
  - nuts
  - grapes
  - hot dog pieces
  - balloons
  - coins
  - small candies or gum
  - raisins
  - popcorn

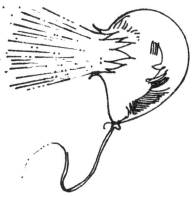

- Children should be supervised while eating and encouraged to sit quietly and chew their food well
- tie knots in plastic bags before throwing them away
- never give babies a pillow
- never place babies on water beds
- be sure your crib meets safety standards and has a large enough mattress; for details, contact your community or public health department or your public health nurse

ELECTRIC SHOCK:

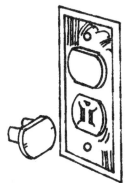

- put covers on all electrical outlets
- use devices to ensure plugs cannot be pulled out of outlets
- keep cords out of sight of small children, but **not** under carpets or mats
- keep electric appliances away from water

Toy Safety

IT'S UP TO YOU:

Supervise children when then are playing with toys. Even though the government and toy companies monitor the safety of toys, it's up to parents to make sure that a toy is:

- used properly (read instructions)
- not broken (inspect regularly)
- right for your child's age

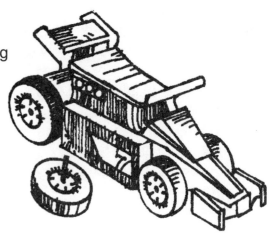

WATCH FOR:

- sharp edges or points
- small pieces that can break off (e.g., wheels, doll's eyes, building blocks)
- plastic wrapping
- balloons
- broken crayon pieces
- small batteries that may be eaten or that are corroded
- adult items that might be toxic (e.g., markers, paint, glue)

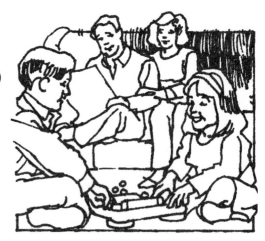

Bicycle Safety

80% of bicycle-related deaths occur because of head injury. All children must wear helmets when riding bikes.

Proper helmets have:

• CSA, ANSI or Snell stickers inside

• adjustable pads and chin straps to ensure the helmet covers the forehead

• a hard outer shell and shock-absorbing inner lining

Children are seldom mature enough to follow basic road rules.

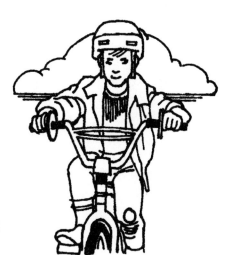

Children Need to Know:

• ride on the right, **with** traffic

• obey all stop signs and red lights

• watch out for and yield to traffic

• watch for right-turning traffic

• children under 12 years of age should walk their bikes through busy intersections

Traffic Safety

CAR SEATS AND RESTRAINTS:

- Car seats must always be placed in the rear seat of the vehicle.
- 35 to 45 percent of infant and toddler car seats are **not** installed or buckled up properly! These children are at high risk of injury.
- You must install the seat according to the manufacturer's instructions. If you don't have these instructions, they can be obtained through CAA or AAA (Canadian or American Automobile Association).
- If you are using a second-hand car seat, you must be sure the seat has never been in an accident.
- Front facing seats for children more than 9 kg (20 pounds) or 66cm (26 inches), must be attached to the vehicle by a tether strap. If you have a vehicle made before 1989 and are unsure where to put the anchor bolt, call the vehicle manufacturer, or CAA or AAA (Canadian or American Automobile Association).

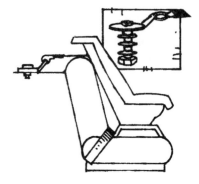

- Be sure to slide the chest clip on the front harness, up to the child's armpit level. Otherwise the child may slide out of the seat in an accident.
- Try not to have bulky winter clothing between your child and the car seat harness. It is very easy for a child in a large bunting bag or snow suit to slip out the top of the harness in an accident. Instead, cut holes through the blankets or snow suit so that the harness straps can be done up inside the outfit, next to the baby's body.

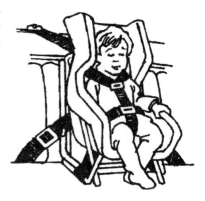

- If your seat belt has a latch that slides freely up and down the strap, you need a locking clip when you install a forward facing car seat. This will stop the seat belt from slowly loosening. This clip is available where car seats are sold.

SAFETY RULES:

Children learn safety rules by watching and doing. Be a good role model:

- stop at corners
- look and listen for traffic
- don't jay walk
- walk on the left, facing traffic
- Practice with your children hundreds of times before you let them cross a street alone.
- Children should not be on the streets and sidewalks after dark. If this cannot be helped, have them wear light colors or, even better, reflective materials or strips.

Water Safety

Drowning is the second leading cause of death in children under 15 years of age.

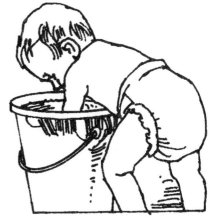

- Never leave children under four alone with water (e.g., beach, pool, bathtub or pail), not even for a few seconds.

- Lifeguards are not supervisors, they provide emergency care. Parents or guardians must provide the required supervision.

- In boats or at the beach, make sure children have approved life jackets or personal flotation devices (PFD).

- A personal flotation device (PFD) must have an official government label saying approved. Children's PFDs should have a crotch strap and be fitted to the child's height and weight.

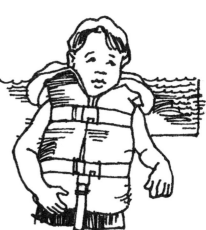

- Water wings and other inflatable toys are **not** safe to use as PFDs.

- Enroll your pre-schooler in swimming lessons to learn swimming skills as well as water safety.

- Be a good example: observe safety rules and wear a life jacket.

Farm Safety

A farm is full of interesting things to see and do, but you must also be careful when enjoying them.

1. Don't allow children to tease animals or stand behind horses or cows. Animals with young may be especially aggressive.

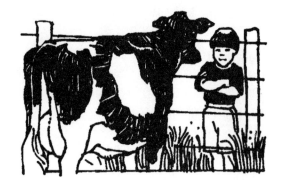

2. Don't go near any machinery that is running. Even if children are not touching machinery, they may slip, trip or have their clothing caught.

3. Ensure that all sharp tools and farm chemicals are safely stored out of reach of children.

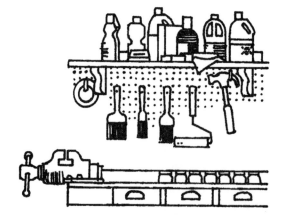

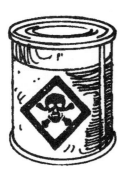

 Keep chemicals in their original containers or clearly label a container if you put a different chemical into it. Children may accidentally drink a poison if it is in a food container.

 Keep children away from areas that have been sprayed with chemicals.

6 Ensure that you and your children have protective goggles when watching welding. Keep children far away from sparks.

NOTES:

References

Adams, Cathrine. 1994. *When Seconds Count ... The Canadian Emergency Treatment Manual.* Edmonton, AB: Emergency Medical Handbooks International Inc.

Advanced Burn Life Support Provider's Manual.

American Academy of Orthopaedic Surgeons. *Rural Rescue and Emergency Care.* 1993. Chicago, IL.

American Academy of Pediatrics. 1994. *Pediatric Advanced Life Support.* Washington, DC: American Heart Association.

American Medical Association. *Handbook of First Aid & Emergency Care.*

Baldwin, Gregory A. 1994. *Handbook of Pediatric Emergencies.* Boston, MA: Little, Brown and Company.

Barkin, Roger M. and Rosin, Peter. 1990. *Emergency Pediatrics: A Guide to Ambulatory Care.* (Third Edition). St. Louis, MO: C.V. Mosby Company.

Berenson, A. (Ed). 1990. *Control of Communicable Diseases in Man.* Washington, DC: APHA.

Bradley, Betty (Ed.). 1994. *The New Baby and Child Care Quick Reference Encyclopedia.* (4th Edition). Toronto, ON: Family Communications Inc.

Canada Safety Council. 1990.

Canadian Injury Prevention Program. *Protect Your Child from Head Injury.*

Canadian Pediatric Society. 1992. *Well Beings.* Toronto, ON: Creative Premises Ltd.

Canadian Red Cross Society. 1988. *Childsafe: A Parent's Guide to First Aid and Safety.* Ottawa, ON.

Caravajal, H.F. and Parks, D.H. 1988. *Burns in Children: Pediatric Burn Management.* Chicago IL: Year Book Medical Publishers Inc.

Charnoff, Dr. Ira. 1994. *Your Child: A Medical Guide.* Lincolnwood, IL: Publications International Ltd.

Children's National Medical Centre. *Safe Kids are No Accident.* Washington DC.

Chung, Stanley M.K. 1986. *Handbook of Pediatric Orthopedics.* New York, NY: Van Nostrand Reinhold Company.

References

Crain, Ellen F.; Geishel, Jeffrey C.; and Gallagher, John E. (Editors). 1992. *Clinical Manual of Emergency Pediatrics.* (Second Edition). New York, NY: McGraw-Hill.

D.S.C. of Saint-Luc Hospital, in Feeding your Child ages 2 to 5. Dairy Bureau of Canada.

DeBolt, Dorothy and Robert. 1994. *Discipline is Love.* Brantford, ON: Independent Order of Foresters.

Disciplining Your Child. 1988. Brantford, ON: Independent Order of Foresters.

Eichelberger, M.R.; Ball, J.W.; Pratsch, G.S. and Runion, E. 1992. *Pediatric Emergencies.* Englewood Cliffs, NJ: Prentice-Hall, Inc.

Farmedic Instructor Manual. New York, NY: Alfred State College.

Foley, Denise; Nechas, Eileen; et al. 1994. *The Doctor's Book of Home Remedies for Children.* Emmaus, PA: Rodale Press.

Gettis, Kagan. *Current Pediatric Therapy.*

Green, M. 1994. *A Sigh of Relief: The First-Aid Handbook for Childhood Emergencies.* New York, NY: Bantam Books.

Grossman, Moses and Dieckman, Ronald A. (Editors). 1991. *Pediatric Emergency Medicine.* Philadelphia, PA: Lippincott Co.

Hart, Dr. Terril H. (Ed). *The Parent's Guide to Baby & Child Medical Care.* Decpharen, MN: Meadowbrooke Press.

Hazinski, M.F. 1992. *Nursing Care of the Critically Ill Child.* St. Louis, MO: Mosby Year Book Inc.

Health and Welfare Canada. 1991. *Sexually Transmitted Diseases.* Ottawa, ON: Supply and Services, Canada.

Health Canada. 1995. *Canada's Food Guide - Focus on Preschoolers.*

Health Canada. *Kids Care.*

Heart and Stroke Foundation of Canada. 1993. *Cardiopulmonary Resuscitation - Basic Rescuer.* Ottawa, ON: Heart and Stroke Foundation of Canada.

Kidd, P. and Stuart, P. 1996. *Emergency Nursing Reference.* St. Louis, MO: Mosby Inc.

Le Francoise, G.R. 1989. *An Introduction to Child Development.* Belmont, C.A.: Wadsworth Publishing Co.

References

Levin, Daniel L. and Morriss, Frances C. 1990. *Essentials of Pediatric Intensive Care.* St. Louis, MO: Quality Medical Publishing Inc.

Lovejoy, Dr. Frederick H. (Editor). 1987. *Boston Children's Hospital - The New Child Health Encyclopedia.*

Merenstein, Gerald B.; Kaplan, David W.; and Rosenberg, Adam A. 1994. *Handbook of Pediatrics.* (17th Edition). Norwalk, CT: Appleton & Lange.

Nelson Textbook on Pediatrics. (13th Edition). Zehrman and Vaughn.

Ontario Physical and Health Education Association and the Canadian Association for Health, Physical Education, Recreation and Dance. 1994. *Vibrant Faces.*

Regina Health District, Community Health Division.

Regina Health District. 1993. *Impetigo.*

Roberts, Kenneth A. 1995. *Manual of Clinical Problems in Pediatrics.* (4th Edition).

Saskatchewan Health. *Baby's First Foods.* Regina, SK: Saskatchewan Health.

Saskatchewan Health. *Feeding Your Baby: The First Year of Life.* Regina SK: Saskatchewan Health

Saskatchewan Health. *The Complete Picture for Children 1 - 5 years.* Regina SK: Saskatchewan Health.

Saskatchewan Health. 1987. *Understanding Depression and Suicide.* Edmonton, AB: Alberta Education.

Sheehy, Susan Budassi. 1992. *Emergency Nursing, Principles and Practice.* (Third Edition). St. Louis, MO: C.V. Mosby, Inc.

The Elementary Safety Book for Children. 1993. Edmonton, AB: Regional Maple Leafe Communications Inc.

Whaley & Wong. *Introduction to Food & Weight Problems.* Toronto, ON: National Eating Disorder Information Centre.

Whaley, Lucille F. and Wong, Donna L. 1995. *Nursing Care of Infants and Children.* (Fifth Edition) St. Louis, MO: Mosby Year Book Inc.

Wood, Dr. Margeret. 1991. *The Baby and Child Care Quick Reference Encyclopedia.* (Volume 2, Issue 1).

Index

E

F

N

HOUSEHOLD HINTS – Money and Time-Saving Ideas for Home and Garden – Revised Edition – 10% more Hints.

From cleaning your chandelier crystals safely in the diswasher, to prolonging the life of your pantihose by freezing them, through numerous cleaning, cooking, gardening, pet, beauty and health tips, *Household Hints* provides useable, useful and sometimes startling solutions to everyday problems. A Canadian best-seller, updated in its seventh printing.

Retail $12.95   144 pages
6" x 9"   50 line drawings   wire coil bound

WORK TIPS – Organizing Strategies for a Productive Worklife
by Patricia Katz

A professional speaker, trainer, consultant and columnist, Patricia combines practical suggestions with humor to help you with professional and business organization time and stress management. Learn how to control paperwork and manage on the run with maximum efficiency.

Retail $14.95   128 pages
6" x 9"   fully illustrated   perfect bound

HOME TIPS – Organizing Strategies for a Streamlined Homelife
by Patricia Katz

Family and household organizational tips are the focus here. Patricia has created a helpful, humorous and practical guide to help you balance housekeeping, family and personal obligations, take care of the essentials, get more out of life and expand your personal choices.

Retail $14.95   128 pages
6" x 9"   fully illustrated   perfect bound

HOUSEHOLD HINTS – Environmental, Energy, Money and Time-Saving Hints for Home and Garden

This "green version" of *Household Hints* provides hundreds of recycling ideas and environmentally friendly alternatives for home and garden, cleaning and maintenance problems. Many of these environmental and energy-conscious hints use low-cost, old-fashioned, common-sense remedies for everyday problems. Your budget and environment will love it.

Retail $9.95   96 pages
6" x 9"   40 line drawings   wire coil bound

A YEAR OF CRAFTS – For Children & Adults
by Geraldine Hartman

Imaginative craft projects, many with seasonal themes, provide year-round pleasure. Each two-page spread features one child's and one adult's craft with photographs and detailed material and assembly instructions. Suitable for age 6 and up.

Retail $12.95   120 pages
6" x 9"   104 black and white plus 32 colored photographs   wire coil bound

CORNERSTONES – An Artist's History of the City of Regina
by William Argan with Pam Cowan

Historic commercial buildings, schools, churches, hotels, theatres and so much more. William Argan's striking illustrations bring the history of Regina alive. A pleasure to read, here is a fascinating look at the business, social, political and cultural cornerstones of Regina.

Retail $15.95   144 pages
6" x 9"   over 150 illustrations   perfect bound

HELPFUL GIFT IDEAS

Children's Medical Emergency Handbook _____x $24.95 = $_____
*Household Hints*_____x $12.95 = $_____
*Household Hints – Environmental*_____x $ 9.95 = $_____
Work Tips – Organizing Strategies for a Productive Worklife _____x $14.95 = $_____
Home Tips – Organizing Strategies for a Streamlined Homelife ___x $14.95 = $_____
A Year of Crafts – For Children & Adults _____x $12.95 = $_____
Cornerstones, An Artist's History of the City of Regina _____x $15.95 = $_____
Shipping and handling charge _____ = $_____3.00____
Subtotal _____ = $_____
In Canada add 7% GST_____(Subtotal x .07) = $_____
Total enclosed_____ = $_____

U.S. and international orders payable in U.S. funds/Prices subject to change.

NAME: _____

STREET:_____

CITY: _____ PROV./STATE _____

COUNTRY _____ POSTAL CODE/ZIP _____

Please make cheque or money order payable to:

THE LEADER-POST CARRIER FOUNDATION INC.
P.O. Box 2020
1964 Park Street
Regina, Saskatchewan, Canada S4P 3G4

For fund raising or volume purchase prices, contact:
THE LEADER-POST CARRIER FOUNDATION INC. at (306) 565-8240

HELPFUL GIFT IDEAS

Children's Medical Emergency Handbook _____x $24.95 = $_____
*Household Hints*_____x $12.95 = $_____
*Household Hints – Environmental*_____x $ 9.95 = $_____
Work Tips – Organizing Strategies for a Productive Worklife _____x $14.95 = $_____
Home Tips – Organizing Strategies for a Streamlined Homelife ___x $14.95 = $_____
A Year of Crafts – For Children & Adults _____x $12.95 = $_____
Cornerstones, An Artist's History of the City of Regina _____x $15.95 = $_____
Shipping and handling charge _____ = $_____3.00____
Subtotal _____ = $_____
In Canada add 7% GST_____(Subtotal x .07) = $_____
Total enclosed_____ = $_____

U.S. and international orders payable in U.S. funds/Prices subject to change.

NAME: _____

STREET:_____

CITY: _____ PROV./STATE _____

COUNTRY _____ POSTAL CODE/ZIP _____

Please make cheque or money order payable to:

THE LEADER-POST CARRIER FOUNDATION INC.
P.O. Box 2020
1964 Park Street
Regina, Saskatchewan, Canada S4P 3G4

For fund raising or volume purchase prices, contact:
THE LEADER-POST CARRIER FOUNDATION INC. at (306) 565-8240